CAREER DIRECTIONS

for

DENTAL HYGIENISTS

Your Guide to Change and Opportunity

By

Regina Dreyer Thomas, RDH

Career Directions Press
171 Highway 34, Holmdel, New Jersey 07733

Career Directions for Dental Hygienists: Your Guide to Change and Opportunity.
Copyright 1992 by Regina Dreyer Thomas. Printed and bound in the United States of America. All rights reserved. No part of this book may be reproduced in any form or by any electronic or mechanical means including information storage and retrieval systems without permission in writing from the publisher, except by a reviewer who may quote brief passages in a review. Published by Career Directions Press, 171 Hwy. 34, Holmdel, NJ 07733. Third edition.

Publisher's Cataloging in Publication
(Prepared by Quality Books Inc.)

Thomas, Regina D.
    Career Directions for dental hygienists : your guide to change
and opportunity / Regina Dreyer Thomas.
        p.   cm.
    ISBN 0-933163-03-7
    1. Dental hygiene—Vocational guidance.   I. Title.
RK60   617.6'01'024
                                                                        QBI91–1338

Library of Congress Catalog Card Number 91–075898
Cover design by Karen Wilson

To My Family

and

Hygiene Buddies

Foreword

Selecting a career 25 years ago was a simple matter for those of us raised in traditional families. Women were expected to raise children and be good homemakers first. They were smart if they had enough education to work if they had to. My family's advice: "get yourself a trade you can fall back on if the man you marry turns out to be an alcoholic." So many of us looked for two- to four-year post-high school programs that would give us a specific skill. Dental hygiene met those criteria.

While many of us may have taken the path that tradition established for us (and considered dental hygiene a "good fallback" or part-time endeavor), there are many more of us who have found dental hygiene to be well worth a lifetime's investment.

Dental hygiene has proven to be a uniquely challenging, diversified and changing career. It is certainly more than a skill and more than a trade. It is an attitude toward dental health care that is valuable in a variety of settings and opportunities. Each one of us has found a way to apply dental hygiene theory and culture in a special way.

Some of us have made traditional clinical practice most untraditional. We have rewritten the way patients are treated, moving away from the routine, cosmetic orientation to a patient-centered, individualized approach to care that integrates the most recent research findings.

Others of us have taken our education and our culture as prevention experts and caregivers to other environments: industry, research, finance, education, administration, patient advocacy and personal entrepeneurship. We have taken the solid basis that dental hygiene provides and used it to create new opportunities for ourselves.

This new edition of *Career Directions for Dental Hygienists* highlights some of the ways we have created new careers for ourselves using dental hygiene as the starting point. The stories included here are inspiring, touching, fun and real. They cameo some of the best and the brightest in dental hygiene—people who have discovered that their personal and professional potential could be realized in a variety of ways.

I invite you to read these stories and enjoy the success; first vicariously and then personally. Let these stories help you make the next step in your career that can help you renew your love for the profession and your zest for daily living. Notice that each person took a risk in order to gain. Each person sought out opportunities, or at least recognized the golden opportunity when it was there to take. They succeeded because they believed they could meet a new challenge and because they prepared for it. Notice also that each person reflects just a little bit of surprise at how well things have turned out.

We can and regularly do achieve beyond the expectations our families and we place upon ourselves when making those first career choices. Writing their stories has undoubtedly helped all the writers feel good about themselves and their achievements.

How does *your* story read? What steps have made *you* feel proud and successful? What might help *you* write a new chapter in your career development? Each of us has a story to be proud of. The key is to continually renew it.

Regina Dreyer Thomas has once again provided us with a book that captures the momentum and spirit of dental hygiene on the move. Thank you, Regina!

Irene R. Woodall, RDH, PhD
Director, Clinical Research and Professional Communications
Vipont Pharmaceutical, Inc.
Fort Collins, Colorado

Table of Contents

Introduction

Have you ever seen a picture of or remember a 1950's hygienist standing chairside by her patient? One dressed in a starched white, long-sleeved skirted uniform, wearing white nylons and oxfords and a purple-banded perky white cap held in place by white bobby pins crossed over each other? That was me.

What I didn't know about scattered radiation, antimicrobial agents, ultrasonic equipment, sitting down, even Gracey curets would fill another book. I vowed to the State Board of Dentistry never to go below the epithelial attachment. My goal was to save the teeth of the world through caries prevention. A thorough prophylaxis, elimination of refined sugars from the diet, topical fluoride applications, and a home care regimen of proper brushing and flossing were what I taught my patients.

I was a graduate of the first class of the then newly-resurrected Fones School of Dental Hygiene in Bridgeport, Connecticut. My pride as my parents watched me being "capped" was exceeded only by the day when my son watched as I capped the students of the school's 25th graduating class a quarter of a century later. Proud to be a dental hygienist then; proud to be a hygienist now.

As I look back on my endeavors, I am caught by the variety of experiences I have had in dental health: clinician in private practice, school dental hygienist, supervisor of a hospital-based public health program, clinical instructor in a school of dental hygiene, training director for a manufacturer of dental products, seminar presenter, writer, publisher, consultant . . . and always with RDH after my name.

Building professional experiences, acquiring degrees, having a family—all are part of a career pattern. And that is the philosophical focus of this book: dental hygiene is a *career*, not a series of jobs in one setting. Private practice is an *option*, not a locked room.

Through this book you will be introduced to over 20 dynamic, achieving RDHs who have taken their skills and abilities and parlayed them into a variety of experiences which are bringing them fulfillment and professional satisfaction; the kind that comes from seeking challenges, then mastering them.

What are their keys to success? How did these people achieve their goals—and why? What is it that motivates them? Perhaps it's the need to accept new challenges in their lives. Perhaps the reasons are as varied as the writers themselves.

As you peruse their stories, assess yourself. See what makes *you* tick; what makes *you* feel proud. (Learn how to do that in the first chapter.)

About the authors. Where did I find them? I am privileged to meet fantastic RDHs through my work with *RDH* magazine, my lectures and through colleagues. (It's called networking.) With few editorial changes, the respective voices are as spoken. I am deeply grateful to each of them for the careful thought and vigor that went into their writings. Their enthusiasm for being a part of dental hygiene comes through loud and clear. We are glad they allowed us to share their histories. The passion, commitment and excitement which govern their lives give credence to our profession and made producing the book a joy.

There were others who had a part in bringing this third edition together. My considerable thanks goes to Laura Albrecht, Carla Beverly, Claudine Paula Drew, Janice Propcheck, Rita Rauzin, Morris Roberts, Denise Sabol, Annette Scheive, Katherine Simons and Karin Wilson. My husband, Neil Thomas, receives my loving gratitude for being there for me. He always is.

I brought *Career Directions for Dental Hygienists* into existence because I believe the continued forward growth of our profession demands a resource devoted exclusively to career opportunities and their successful management. I hope that premise, reflected in the writings, meets your expectations and fills your needs in reaching your own career goals in dental health care.

Upward and onward!

Regina Dreyer Thomas, RDH
Editor & Publisher

"MANY TIMES IDEAS GROW BETTER WHEN TRANSPLANTED FROM ONE MIND TO ANOTHER."
—*Oliver Wendell Holmes*

Looking at Yourself First

Linda Rubinstein-DeVore *is an associate professor and director of the degree completion program at the University of Maryland Dental School in Baltimore. She lectures and counsels dental hygiene students and practitioners on how to create personal and professional growth patterns.*

Looking at Yourself

You are anxious to begin exploring this book. You have already flipped through the pages and a few of the chapter titles have caught your eye. Some of the career paths described by our colleagues sound exciting. You are hoping that at least one of these descriptions will give you an idea for the right directions for your career.

Wait a minute. Before you look at what other dental hygienists have done to achieve success and satisfaction in their careers, you need to spend some time thinking about yourself. Do you know what you are looking for in your profession? Do you have a good understanding of what makes you happy in your work life? Have you thought about how your personal and professional lives fit together?

While it may seem easier to start by reading about what others have done and analyzing yourself later, career counselors suggest that this is not the best approach. You need to gain an understanding of yourself first so that you can evaluate the options others have chosen.

Consider this analogy. You are on your way home from work and are rather hungry. You don't have a shopping list with you. You know the combination of hunger and no list is dangerous in the supermarket, but you stop at the store anyway. You end up spending more than you should have on items you really didn't need or want; they seemed appealing at the time. I agree, this is no big deal. You will shop again in a few more days, and certainly you haven't spent your life savings.

The search for a new career direction, which may involve a job change, is a far more serious matter. Yet many of us go about it with little more thought and planning than for the impromptu trip to the store. We are hungry for something different, but we don't know exactly what will satisfy. Plunging into a job search may seem like a good plan. Not true. Our professional lives are too important to leave to such a haphazard approach.

Let me suggest a more systematic plan. In its most simple form, career planning involves gaining an understanding of yourself, writing down your goals, exploring the available options for achieving your goals, and establishing and implementing an action plan. All of this is done in the context of your overall life plan. Career goals and personal goals must fit together.

Simple, ha! This sounds too complex and tedious. Self-assessment . . . written goals . . . action plans . . . is all this really necessary? YES! It will be worth the effort.

In my position as director of a baccalaureate degree completion program, I have counseled hundreds of dental hygienists in search of new career directions. Many of them are returning to school to expand their career options. They want to know what new opportunities will be available to them after graduation. In our discussions, I tell them what some of our graduates are doing, but mostly I help them focus on themselves. What do they like about dental hygiene and the practice experiences they've had? What don't they like? What are their special skills, talents and interests? What are their goals?

Ultimately, the search for new career options is not so much about what others have done, but about what *you* want to do. Our colleagues tell us about the choices they've made and how they've advanced professionally; yet each of us has to develop in our own way. Each of us gains satisfaction from a unique combination of experiences in education, work and leisure activities.

Before you read the autobiographical essays in this book, take some time for self-analysis. It isn't difficult. It may be fun! Most importantly, you may reach a level of self-awareness that will give you confidence to embark on your own new career direction, one that will be right for *you.*

Take out some paper or write in this book. First think, then write your answers to the following questions.

Setting Your Goals

1. What would you like to accomplish within a year?

2. What would you like to accomplish within five years?

3. On a scale of 1 to 10 (highest value), how important to you is each of the goals identified above? Based on this rating, identify a priority for each goal and put a circle around the number.

Looking Within

1. What are your ten best skills, talents and special interests?

2. What three things do you like *most* about your current job?

Your previous job?

3. What three things do you like *least* about your current job?

Your previous job?

4

4. What strengths (persistence, tenacity, assertiveness, etc.) do you have that will help you achieve your goals?

5. What weaknesses or constraints (personal, family, financial, educational, etc.) do you have that will inhibit achievement of your goals?

6. Which of these weaknesses or constraints can you change? How?

Exploring the Options

1. Now read about what other hygienists have done. When you've finished this book, talk to colleagues and read current journals to learn more about opportunities for dental hygienists. Evaluate what others have done in the context of your self-analysis. Identify positions which maximize things you like most in your work environment and minimize those you like least.

2. Look around you and consider settings where you might have something to offer. You can *create* new job opportunities; others have done it.

3. Consider whether it is possible to achieve your career goals in your present job. Don't overlook possibilities for change in your current practice situation.

4. Write down the options that appeal to you the most.

Developing an Action Plan

1. Write out each goal and a timetable (date) for completing it.

2. If you need additional education (continuing or a formal degree), make plans to attain it. Obtain appropriate catalogues, talk to academic advisors, make the decision to begin *now*. Write down your short- and long-term educational plans.

3. If you are ready to seek a new position, brush up your job interviewing skills, update your résumé and begin. This book and many others available in bookstores and libraries will provide guidance for the process of an effective job search.

Evaluating Your Progress

1. At six month and yearly intervals, evaluate your progress toward achieving your goals. Write down your achievements and revise your plans if necessary.

Six Months

End of First Year

Remember, self-assessment and planning should be ongoing activities throughout your life. If you want to achieve your potential (and who among us does not), you need to take charge. Start with a realistic look at yourself and plan for your own successful career direction. Good luck!

Suggested References

Bolles, Richard N., *The Three Boxes of Life*. Berkeley, CA: Ten Speed Press, 1981.

Bolles, Richard N., *What Color is Your Parachute?* Berkeley, CA: Ten Speed Press, 1991.

RDH in Public Health

Preface

Loosely called "people's health," the American Academy of Dental Public Health defines public or community health as ". . . concerned with the dental health education of the public, with applied dental research and with the administration of group dental care programs, as well as the prevention and control of dental diseases on a community basis."

Such a definition literally shouts for dental hygiene to lead the way. Aren't RDHs uniquely trained to focus on prevention, health promotion and education, the bulwark of most public health programs?

Consider the possibilities: we can conduct dental health education programs for all age groups and socioeconomic levels, perform screenings, design, implement and monitor surveys, refer, manage fluoride mouthrinse programs or spearhead water fluoridation activity, apply fissure sealants, develop resource materials, co-promote with professional groups, organizations and health agencies, write grants . . . the list is virtually endless.

The next three entries are from three dental hygienists who have allied themselves with community dental health settings as a means of career growth. They tell us what makes their work so interesting, challenging and fulfilling.

RDH in the Public Schools

Susan Goldner *outlines her success as a community dental health educator.*

How I Started

My present career position came easy. I was, pardon the expression, "made an offer I couldn't refuse." Since 1984 I have been the dental coordinator/administrator for a county public health department in central New York State.

I had spent ten years in private practice in three different offices working either full time or part time, depending on my family's needs. I came to dental hygiene by way of dental assisting.

One week after graduating with an associate's degree in elementary education (planning initially to pursue a bachelor's degree), I got married. Two children followed within the next few years, yet at age 24 I wanted to work part time and do something of my own. I applied for and was hired as a dental assistant. It was in this situation that I found the interest and career I wanted to pursue: dental hygiene.

Luckily a nearby community college offered a dental hygiene program. Tuition was affordable. I could commute and because I already had an associate's degree, I could organize a good schedule of only dental hygiene courses and clinic work. I loved all of it . . . the classes, the instructors, my fellow classmates.

The two years flew by and I landed the first job I applied for. It's my belief that the enthusiasm I have for dental hygiene got it for me. I loved the work and the patients and the money was fine for a woman right out of school in 1974 and now divorced.

Dental hygiene was always good to me. I could take time off if my children had a school play, brownie pinning or special event. I learned a lot about my community and met all kinds of people of different ages, with interesting needs and philosophies.

One day I answered an ad in the paper for a Head Start Dental Hygienist. Several hygienists applied, but my associate's degree in elementary education pushed me to the front. Although the position was part time, it had so many different aspects: writing for the newletter, writing the center's dental health plans, doing workshops with staff and parents, and, of course, the children. Even at age four their needs were tremendous.

I called the local health department and asked permission to use their dental clinic (which they maintained but used only on a very limited basis). This enabled me to let the children experience the dental environment first-hand. For most, this was their first exposure to dentistry. I could then screen and categorize follow-up care as needed.

Along with the Head Start staff, I found many innovative ways to get funding so that these children's dental needs would be met, and to help their parents get a better knowledge of dentistry. I was becoming known around town!

Along with my main job, I also started to work part time at a local rehabilitation center (350 patients; 85% geriatric) doing screenings, caring for dentures and partials, and scheduling exams and follow-up care with the dentist.

So, I held three part-time jobs in 1984, all varied with flexible hours—a real must for a parent of two teenagers! I was doing this when I got "the offer I couldn't refuse." Because of my varied jobs, the director of the county health department noticed me and my enthusiasm for my work. He had a new position available. Was I interested? Even though my experience with public health at the time was limited to one required course in school and a visit to the dental section of the public health department in a metropolitan area, I felt my experience and style and knowledge of the community would be an asset. Besides, I really wanted to work for one place and receive one paycheck.

What the Position Entailed

The position, director/coordinator of a new program funded by the Dental Bureau of the New York State Department of Health, would require the person to develop and implement a dental education/screening program for the schools in our county. A dental sealant program was planned for the future.

This meant seven districts, 16,600 students and lots of miles needing to be covered. I spoke with a fellow hygiene graduate. We started to throw ideas back and forth and network a few classroom programs. She was enjoying the concept and soon was part of the new dental education team.

We started in the spring and put together a program for targeted grades K, 2, 5, 8 and 11. Throughout the summer I worked on budgets, scheduling and supplies and learned as much as I could about dental public health. Our program was going to be unique. Prevention was the key, with follow-up referrals made to the home schools.

Today, after many starts, stops and changes, we have seven years of credibility leading the way. From the beginning I realized there would be no rigid parameters to restrict my development of the program. Yes, of course good dentistry and hygiene practices would be paramount. Yes, children, parents and school staff would be educated. Yes, supervision would be provided. But the bottom line was, this was mine to develop and press on with. A most appealing goal.

The Program's Growth

With my colleague at my side, we gently eased into a program of teaching, screening and sealing teeth. We developed permission slips, distribution lists, personnel contracts, travel routes, logistics, and hundreds of other items you wouldn't believe were necessary until you tried to start a program like this.

We've done more than just educate, screen and seal. We've served as resource personnel and public health educators. Community health fairs, teachers' workshops, prenatal classes, Head Start programs, parent workshops, the community dental advisory board, the Women, Infant and Children (WIC) program . . . these are just some of the organizations and institutions we have contributed to. With a well-trained staff of two hygienists, one assistant and one secretary, our capability to fulfill the original "charter" flows smoothly onward.

Our greatest credibility is the rapport and grass-roots level support we have *earned* with the staff at all seven school districts. Administrators and teachers alike have been extremely supportive of our programs, time management and resource materials. Their encouragement has also made the children aware of the importance of the program.

My proudest thoughts at this time are that the offer I couldn't refuse has brought me to a point where I can make a difference. This is very important to me. I look forward to servicing the needs of the children in my county with continuous dedication, as well as viewing my career with great personal satisfaction. I love it!

13

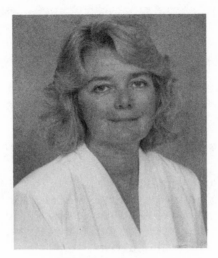

Susan Goldner

RDH in a Family Clinic

Daughn B. Thomas *discusses her multi-faceted roles in a neighborhood family health care clinic and in the military.*

In the Beginning

As a child, I always wanted to be a teacher. When I finished high school, I knew I wanted to be a physical education instructor, but my mother had other plans for me. She wanted me to be a nurse. Even though I attended nursing school, I did not apply myself and dropped out. My mother was very angry with me and told me I'd have to go to secretarial school. I finished it, but hated the work. I knew there had to be something better out there for me.

I finally decided to do something in the medical field. But what? One day while commuting to my job I saw an ad on the train for dental assisting. I thought, "That's in the medical field, and only a small part of the body. How hard can it be to learn?" I found a school located near where I worked, went evenings for a year, and graduated.

Being an Assistant

I liked being a dental assistant but after six years, became bored. I found a job as an assistant supervisor where I had more responsibility. It was in this office that I became aware of dental hygiene. There were four dental hygienists employed there. As I watched them work, I thought, "Why can't I do that?" I spoke to them about the profession and the schools they attended. They were very encouraging. I also spoke to my director and he helped me get into a school.

I had never before thought seriously about going to college. (How was I going to be a teacher—my childhood dream—without it?) The idea scared me. Would I be able to do it? With some persuasion from my boss and a few phone calls, I went to the college to find out what the process entailed. I took the entrance exam, passed the grade and entered hygiene school.

Back to School

School was rough for me. Classes were 8 AM to 4:30 PM. Since I had to work to support myself, I worked in the evenings from 5 to 8 PM and every Saturday from 8 AM to 4 PM. I had to study harder than the others with less time to do so. Two and one-half years with no real social life. If I did go out, my books went with me. It was a very intense time with lots of tears but also lots of laughter. I didn't think I would make it but I did. I graduated first in my class.

Job Hunting Again

Disappointment came. After all that sweat and tears, I found out how difficult it was for me, a black woman, to get a job in private practice. When they saw this young-looking black female walk through their door, I knew from the look on their faces I didn't have a chance in a million to get the job. My dental assisting experience and class ranking didn't seem to matter. The job was either taken or "we have to interview other people." Of course, I was not the one chosen. This even happened with black dentists. They asked me "why not be an assistant instead of a hygienist?" and never explained their reasons for saying this. I would walk out of the interview dumbfounded. I couldn't understand why the black dentist wouldn't hire me or just wanted me to assist. Needless to say, I was totally confused.

I was now out of school for four months, running out of money and needed a job. I took a position with an oral surgeon as an assistant. Meanwhile, I applied, took the test, and joined the Army Reserves.

The Military and Dental Hygiene

Back to blood, sweat and tears. Basic training was very difficult but I survived and graduated with honors and letters. Since I had an associate's degree, I received the rank of private first class when I left basic training.

I went into a medical unit where my job was managing personnel records. I then took the course in dental assisting and received my next rank. To advance quickly, I switched to the dental field, my real interest. After taking innumerable courses, I was in the dental unit.

I now have the rank of staff sargeant. I teach in the dental assisting course, do clinical dental hygiene, teach prevention and take medical histories. Other times I am in charge of the clinic floor. When I am not chairside, supervising or teaching, I perform my other military duties. All this is done in a military installation one weekend each month except for the two weeks I am on active duty. I now have 13 years in the Reserves.

Shifting Goals

After basic training, I worked in two clinics, tried private practice but only stayed three months. The prejudice was back again. I applied for and took the exam for a position with the City of New York. I was also attending college and earned a B.A. in community health. My interest in teaching was still there, but I needed a master's degree. I enrolled in a master's program and obtained an MPH. I work for the Department of Health and Hospitals in a neighborhood family health care clinic in the Bronx, one of New York City's five boroughs as a dental hygienist and infection control officer.

What I Do

Ninety percent of my time is spent in clinical hygiene. My patients are drawn from all countries and religions. My work is very interesting and I see many abnormalities. Since I see the patients first, I do an extensive medical history, chart, set up my treatment plan, educate, apply fluorides or sealants, do prophys, refer to generalists or specialists.

I am an infection control officer the other ten percent of my time. How this came about is very interesting. I was on the Infection Control Committee for nearly three years. I took the minutes, kept the regulations on file and worked with the inspectors when they came. When the dental director, who was chairman of the committee left, he suggested to administration that I run the committee. This didn't sit too well at first with the physicians and other committee members. (This clinic combines all medical and dental specialties within the facility.) At the first meeting I conducted, I discussed the situation with the members. The meeting ran so well that at the end of it, I could see in their faces and attitudes there would be no problems. I think top administration really wanted a doctor to be in charge, but when they realized I have an MPH, have proven capable, and am formally trained in infection control procedures, they asked me to continue as chair.

This position entails seeing that every employee in the facility is inoculated against hepatitis and measles and tested for TB once a year; reporting needle sticks and other accidents; overseeing environmental conditions throughout the clinic; keeping up with OSHA regulations; and working with the Safety Committee which I am also on.

As infection control officer, it is my responsibility to oversee sterilization and asepsis in the dental clinic. I run tests on the sterilizers, make sure that everyone is using the Centers for Disease Control universal precautions, that there's a place for sharps disposal, that every operator is gloved, masked and gowned with safety glasses in place.

With my hands in so many pies, boredom at work is definitely not an issue.

Private vs Public

Private practice isn't good for me. I don't seem to get along with that setting and the patients. Besides, there's really no challenge.

The city job is exciting. I've seen all sorts of abnormalities, tongue and lip disorders, mouth cancers, extensive periodontitis and periodontosis. I can see improvements in my patients from my hard work. It's rewarding to see patients like the way their mouths look where they didn't before. They are very vocal in their appreciation and interested in education and prevention. Most don't have to be reminded to keep their recall appointments.

In working for the city there is less salary than in private practice; however, you do get a small percentage raise every year. The benefits are excellent: no malpractice insurance, low cost medical benefits, free or no cost prescriptions, 11 to 13 holidays off, accumulated sick time, retirement benefits, pension, vacation time, flexibility, etc. I am able to juggle time for school, teaching and my military duties.

Working in the public sector is good for me and my mental being, but it's not for everyone. It depends on your needs, desires and how you wish to achieve your goals.

The Association

In between all the work and studying, I joined the New York City component of the American Dental Hygienists' Association. I became involved and soon was on the board and a delegate to the state. Before I knew it, I became chair of the membership committee on the state level. I was recommended and thought it would be a new challenge for me. On the city level, I've worked my way up so that I am now president of the New York City component.

I also applied for and was accepted as a charter member of the Academy of Dental Hygiene. One day I'll be a Fellow in the Academy. I'm also very near to securing that teaching position I've been working toward.

For me, dental hygiene has been very challenging—but exhausting. Yet I love it. You can, too. You can go as far as you want with it. The more education you have, the more doors will open for you.

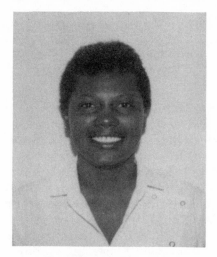

Daughn B. Thomas

RDH and the Homebound

Ellen S. Matje *has formed her career as an administrator within the construct of a grants-funded program for the elderly and medically compromised.*

I had been practicing clinical dental hygiene for 11 years when I was approached by a dental hygiene professor about a position as administrator/faculty supervisor for a new, homebound training and treatment program. The local dental hygiene school had just received a large start-up grant from a private foundation. The responsibilities of the position would be primarily to train senior dental hygiene students to treat frail elderly and medically compromised patients. Since it was a new program, the job would also entail planning the program, developing special care curriculum modules, and being responsible for a large budget. Three staff members would be working on the above activities under my supervision; one hygienist who would supervise rotations at a junior college at a large city, one hygienist who would work out of the state health department coordinating schedules between dentists, faculty and patients, as well as develop the patient pool; one part-time secretary.

My Background

Though disgruntled about the inadequate compensation I had received from employers over the years, I was not at all burned out in clinical dental hygiene. I had worked in various clinical positions in periodontal and general offices, as well as instruct part-time at a dental hygiene school. At the time the offer was made, I was working in a general practice and enjoyed the client/provider relationships I had formed. My abilities were respected and I enjoyed managing the periodontics in the practice. In the '80s, I had completed a two-year expanded functions program in periodontics.

Throughout my undergraduate education and career, I always enjoyed working with special patients: the elderly, developmentally disabled, medically compromised, physically disabled, etc. I was very comfortable with those patients and felt I had innate skill in this area.

20

Starting Over

Though feeling somewhat ambivalent about changing positions, I listened to the ensuing plans and applied for the position. If things were meant to be—this was! I was the only applicant! I jumped head-first into the position and found myself in charge of curriculum development, program planning, balancing a large budget and supervising three other employees. I quickly became oriented to the academic/adminstrative world, and was glad that I had an extensive writing background from my undergraduate education. As a team, the two coordinators and I wrote a quality assurance and procedure manual, designed the program format and created evaluation forms. We attended the University of Washington's DECOD graduate program (Dental Education for the Care of the Disabled), and ordered thousands of dollars' worth of portable equipment and, in general, geared up to begin taking students on rotations to see homebound patients in nursing homes, private homes and sheltered workshops.

Personal Impact

What I did not anticipate was how the new career direction would impact upon my personal life. The new position and tremendous responsibilities boosted my self-esteem considerably. I found the confidence to make major changes in my personal life. One colleague said I transformed from an old woman to a young, vibrant woman overnight. Chronic allergies, insomnia, ulcer symptoms and a bit of extra weight disappeared.

What Homebound Care is Like

Working with the special needs population offers unique challenges, often spur-of-the-moment decisions. In Arizona, homebound patients are required to have been examined within six months of any dental hygiene care (which can be delivered without the direct supervision of a dentist). The team approach to care is very useful. I accompany the dentist as well as the students on visits to homebound clients. The dentist and I discuss the dental hygiene needs of the client, then he writes a total care treatment plan for hygiene and basic dental services.

We have altered our own expectations for patients' dental health to bring them more in line with the health, background and wishes of

21

the patients and their families. Often treatment plans are extremely simple. The student's goal can be to help make a patient's mouth feel more comfortable—quickly. I tell students that the secret to treatment planning for this population is to prioritize the clients' needs and plan treatment accordingly. A compromised patient's stamina can mean no more than 15 minutes of working time. We often deal with years of neglect, inappropriate patient behavior and bad smells. Unique challenges, such as communicating with a non-English-speaking client who is also hard-of-hearing and blind, certainly make our days interesting! Nursing homes seem to refer late-stage Alzheimer cases to us, and these clients can be unresponsive and combative.

Even considering the challenges, the rewards and variety of homebound delivery keep me dedicated. The elderly population is very diverse. This diversity is derived from years of life experience; they defy stereotypes. I have gained from the strength of a 90-year-old woman who outlived all her friends and relatives.

Working with the homebound population means giving extra attention, sometimes crying with an elderly man who feels lonely when it is time for us to leave. Developmentally disabled indivduals are fun to work with but they can be unpredictable, demanding flexibility from the provider. I find that it is crucial to the success of visits to discover background information about each client, such as likes and dislikes. Sheltered workshops often have data sheets that are helpful. Some clients are frightened by loud noises or become violent if certain words are mentioned; others do fine during a dental procedure if someone holds their hand. Others will agree with everything that is asked, even if the questions are conflicting. Developmentally disabled individuals are sensitive to the provider's tone of voice and body language so I encourage students to stay relaxed. TLC is standard protocol.

Skills Needed

There are several skills needed to be successful in homebound dental hygiene. It is necessary to prioritize treatment according to the patient's dental needs, medical condition, stamina and individual wishes. A medically compromised patient can rarely handle root planing, but it is impressive to see how gingivae improve after simpler treatment, such as a quick debriding.

A sense of creativity in problem-solving is needed, such as how to position comfortably to provide care to patients in bed. Good judgement skills help in determining when to delay or modify treatment. I have canceled an appointment because an elderly patient didn't feel well. Two days later the patient died! People in terminal condition due to illnesses like cancer or Parkinson's disease often have fulminating candida infections a week or two before they die. I interpret this as a grave sign.

Efficiency is crucial. Because stress reduction means very short appointments, scaling needs to be quick and effective. A current knowledge of oral medicine and emergency procedures is needed. One should know how to do wheelchair transfers and be able to judge when and when not to attempt them.

How to Get Started

For anyone interested in starting a homebound program, I believe the most important piece of equipment is a good light source, one with a long reach and adjustments at several angles. Aseptico and Mobile Dental Equipment are two companies manufacturing good portable lights.

Most of the instruments and supplies that are needed can be carried in a medium-size plastic bin. I save sample sizes of soap, mouthwash and disinfectant to refill. Disposable cups (one for rinsing, one for spitting) and plenty of gauze can be used instead of an evacuation system. Hygiene care can be delivered simply by using porte polishers.

I wouldn't recommend buying a lot of portable equipment until carefully checking to find out what others are using and how reliable the equipment is. It's helpful to start out with only the basic items until you discover what exactly you need for the population being served. A reclining chair is fine as a dental chair (just cover with a large plastic bag); hospital beds can be positioned conveniently. Many nursing homes have reclining wheelchairs.

Finding patients is not too difficult. Nursing homes' social workers are good contacts for finding out what services are already offered. Most counties offer community services to the elderly, such as meals on wheels. Companies that supply home health care items such as oxygen and hospital beds are good contacts. Catholic and Jewish social service agencies offer services to the homebound population.

The homebound program I manage is funded well enough to allow us to offer our services free of charge to our clients. To be honest, if we charged a fee that was high enough to cover costs, most of our clients couldn't afford it. Travel and setup time is considerable. Homebound is best considered a practice builder. Family and nursing home staff are so impressed by visiting dentists and hygienists, they often refer friends and family members.

I feel dental providers should provide services to their clients who become homebound or are unable to travel. Local associations could provide lights and portable equipment to care for their infirm clients in their homes. Dental professionals always feel good about themselves when they make the extra effort to provide care to those who would otherwise not receive it.

Salaries and Benefits

My salary is more representative of an administrative university scale than a provider of homebound services. In fact, I am tied to the university's pay scale. Even if the foundations would like to pay me more, they can't. I don't make a higher salary than local private practice clinicians make, but my income tax forms reflect a higher and more steady income. University benefits add 35 percent to the value of my salary, and I am still paid when I am sick or on vacation.

The Good and the Bad Sides

I love exposing students to "dentistry in a drum." There is no substitute for the hands-on training received from working with clients who can't visit a conventional clinic. It's valuable to see the clients' environs and really feel their poverty and loneliness. One can learn so much about different medical conditions when providing services to clients who exhibit the signs and symptoms that are listed in textbooks. Students always feel they gain from the experience, though some are more comfortable than others.

The downside to my position is that the homebound program has been funded through private foundation grants, and grants run out. It is very stressful to be employed with soft money.

The program started with a three-year grant. After depletion of those funds, I was awarded another grant from another foundation to maintain the program for another year and a half. I am again looking for funds to support the program. Even if I am lucky to receive multi-year funding, it takes a year or two to receive additional funds. Consequently, I am always searching for money and worrying about whether or not the program will continue. However, I love my work so much, even after five years, I will maintain the efforts it takes to enable it to continue. I am glad I accepted the position that no one else wanted.

24

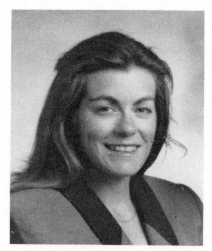

Ellen S. Matje

Dental Hygiene Jobs in the Federal Service

Working for Uncle Sam

According to the U.S. Government's Office of Personnel Management, there are approximately 385 full-time dental hygiene positions in the Federal service, 26 of which are non-clinical community health dental hygiene jobs. This kind of job is gotten through special screening of qualified applicants. A bachelor's degree is required.

Hygienists working for Uncle Sam can be employed by any one of five major agencies: the Veterans Administration (this unit alone employs near 40 percent), Departments of the Army, Navy, Air Force and Health and Human Services (the Indian Health Service comes under this category).

The Department of the Army is the largest employer of the Uniformed Services (does not include RDHs already in the military). The Air Force and Navy have far fewer positions and those only in hospitals.

The title "Dental Hygienist" is used for all positions involving work of a clinical nature, including those assigned duties related to research, teaching, or the performance of dental hygiene expanded functions.

Actually, those RDHs employed in a federal hospital setting such as the VA find their work more interesting than when previously employed in the private sector. Their patients usually have interrelated medical and dental problems, a condition adding to the complexity of their work and offering more challenges. They often find themselves members of a large medical/dental team with a distinct voice in comprehensive treatment planning. Consequently, the turnover rate for these jobs is relatively low. (Look under "Resources" in the back of this book for locations of VA hospitals.)

Job Opportunities

In the past, there have been more job openings for clinical dental hygiene positions than there were dental hygienists to fill them. This situation has changed claims RDH Linda McDaniels Rohrer, president of the only agency specializing in placing full- and part-time RDHs in military dental clinics nationwide.

"We've placed many, many hygienists," she says, "and forecast placing an even greater number in the near future since new contracts are opening up all the time." Such a service can be a boon to RDHs who are relocating or whose spouses are being transferred. In fact, Rohrer points out, many of her clients are military spouses. (See

Dental Power ad in the back of the book. A full listing of dental clinics on military installations is under "Resources.")

Qualifications

Licensure in any state, territory or the District of Columbia is acceptable to Uncle Sam. This means a relocating RDH won't have to go through the trauma and delay of preparing for and retaking state boards—a put-off to many and frequently a reason for leaving hygiene.

In the Federal service, General Service (GS) dental hygienists are paid based on the grade of the position they hold. This grade is set according to the evaluation of the complexity and responsibility of the duties performed. (See next four pages for detailed description of duties.)

For example, Step 1 of the entry level GS-5 paid nearly $17,000 in 1991, going up to over $22,000 for Step 10. (Each grade level has 10 steps.) A spanking new graduate would be qualified to handle the duties outlined for that position.

The GS-6, Step 5 level paid $21,443 in 1991. This person has more patient education and dental staff training responsibilities in addition to working on more advanced perio and postsurgical patients.

Working on a GS-7 level, the highest classification for a staff hygienist, a Step 10 RDH earned nearly $28,000 in 1991. This position has more responsibilities such as lecturing to various patient groups, working with the medical staff, and performing advanced prophylactic and preventive dental procedures in the treatment of patients with related medical and dental problems.

Bear in mind that even though pay scales are lower than in the private sector (although periodically adjusted for cost of living), the benefits are outstanding. The Federal service offers job security, retirement, occupational health and life insurance, and vacation and sick leave. Furthermore, there isn't quite as much pressure to produce by the clock. This permits the hygienist to spend more time in actual treatment and education of the patient.

Dental Hygienist, GS-5

Duties

Serves as a dental hygienist responsible for administering oral prophylaxis, treating abnormal gum conditions, and instructing patients in oral health care.

—Performs complete oral prophylaxis including the following: seats and drapes patients; applies disclosing solution to the teeth; performs supragingival and subgingival scaling using cavitron and scalers to remove calculus deposits, accretions, and stains; polishes teeth using bristle brushes, rubber cups, polishing strips, and prophylactic paste; and applies topical fluorides and other anticariogenic agents. Cleans and polishes removable dental appliances worn by patients.

—Examines patient's oral cavity including the mouth, throat, and pharynx, and records condition of the teeth and surrounding tissues. Refers patients to the dentist who have abnormalities such as cavities, defective fillings, suspicious growths, or periodontal disease. Applies desensitizing agents and other topical agents to treat abnormalities such as gingivitis and Vincent's infection.

—Instructs patients, individually and in groups, in proper oral hygiene care using materials such as teeth models, displays, slides, toothbrushes, dental floss, disclosing tablets, mirrors, and phase microscope. Demonstrate proper techniques of brushing, flossing, and use of necessary perio aids and explains the common causes of tooth decay and its relationship to general diet. Instructs nurses and nursing assistants in oral health care techniques for bedridden, handicapped, disabled, and chronically ill patients.

—Takes, develops, and mounts oral X-rays including bite wing, panoramic and periapical. Interprets X-rays to determine areas of calculus deposits and periodontal involvement, the relationship of the teeth, etc. Selects and arranges X-rays as teaching devices for viewing by patients.

—Records the number of patients treated and type of treatment administered. Checks and maintains instruments to insure working condition. Cleans, sharpens, and sterilizes instruments.

Dental Hygienist, GS-6

Duties

Serves as a dental hygienist responsible for providing routine and advanced prophylactic and therapeutic dental care to postsurgical and periodontal patients.

—Upon referral from the dentist, examines patient's teeth and surrounding tissues to determine extent of abnormal condition requiring treatment. Records a history of each patient to determine if systemic conditions are present which may alter standard treatment. Plans dental hygiene treatment and series of appointments in accordance with existing conditions.

—Performs oral prophylaxis and provides therapeutic care in cases of acute gingivitis and periodontal disease using a variety of scalers and ultrasound equipment. Applies prescribed medicines to gums in cases of excess bleeding. When necessary, under the direction and supervision of the dentist performs deep scaling, root planing and subgingival curettage; takes intraoral impressions for the preparation of study models, smooths and polishes rough edges of restorations; places temporary fillings, administers local anesthesia; and places and removes rubber dams.

—In cases of periodontal surgery performs dressing removal, suture removal, irrigation, and dressing application. Provides therapeutic instruction to patient in the home care phase of treatment adapting instructions, oral hygiene aids and techniques to the individual situation. Teaches patients specialized techniques such as use of interproximal brushes, bridge threaders, and disclosing agents.

—Sets up and maintains a patient recall system to insure continuous, close follow-up treatment for each patient involved in the dental program. Provides instructions using demonstrations and audio-visual aids in the use and care of dental prosthesis, nutritional guidance, and need for daily hygiene care to prevent further dental disease and infections.

—Takes, develops and interprets intraoral and extraoral X-rays to determine areas of calculus deposits and periodontal involvement. Selects and arranges X-rays for special use in educating and motivating the patient.

—Provides dental hygiene instruction and training to other dental service personnel and participates in dental staff meetings and programs.

Dental Hygienist, GS-7

Duties

Serves as a dental hygienist responsible for performing advanced prophylactic and preventive dental procedures in the treatment of patients with related medical and dental problems.

—Completes preliminary dental examinations on new dental service patients. The hygienist reviews patient's medical and dental history for evidences of past and present conditions such as medical illnesses and use of drugs which may complicate or alter dental hygiene treatment; examines the teeth and surrounding tissues for evidences of plaque and periodontal disease and charts findings; inspects the mouth and throat for evidence of disease such as oral cancer; interprets routine X-rays to identify tooth structures, calculus, and abnormalities such as cavities and deep periodontal pockets. Refers abnormalities such as cavities, traumatic occlusion, and suspicious lesions to the dentist. Prepares dental hygiene treatment plans for patient including assessment of the problem, type of oral hygiene care required, and the sequence of appointments needed to complete treatment.

—Performs a complete oral prophylaxis on ambulatory and non-ambulatory patients. Performs deep subgingival scaling, root planing, and curettage under local anesthesia. Polishes the teeth and applies stannous fluoride for hypersensitivity and caries prevention. Gives home care instructions to patients after curettage. Provides bedside prophylactic treatment using specialized procedures for comatose patients, neurosurgical patients, and other types of nonambulatory patients.

—In postoperative care of oral surgery and periodontal surgery patients, performs suture removal, changes dressings, applies topical anesthetics, and provides home care instructions. In oral cancer patients, takes impressions for construction of mouth guards, applies fluoride using tray technique, and maintains recall system for careful follow-up of each patient. Educates patient on need for daily oral health and fluoride treatment.

—Assists the dentist by making repairs and adjustments to the teeth by smoothing rough edges of restorations, removing overhanging margins of fillings, reducing sharp edges of fractured teeth, polishing and finishing amalgam restorations, and inserting temporary fillings in teeth.

—Instructs patients at chairside in oral hygiene, brushing and flossing techniques, and periodontal aids which increase the amount of stimulation to the teeth. Plans and adapts instructions in home care techniques, tailoring them to the oral hygiene needs and oral problems of individual patients. Explains to patients the causes of periodontal disease and tooth decay, and the importance of diet as it relates to oral and systemic health.

—Regularly instructs nurses and nursing assistants in the proper techniques of oral hygiene to be applied to the bedridden, handicapped, disabled and chronically ill patient. Presents lectures and demonstrations in oral health care to various patient groups such as diabetics, hemodialysis patients, and drug or alcohol dependent patients, using slides, denture models, toothbrushes, charts, and other dental education materials.

—Exposes, develops and processes radiographs on patients including bite wing, periapical and panoramic X-rays. Adjusts voltage, amperage, and timing of X-ray equipment. Selects type of radiograph that will be necessary for patient's mouth. Positions film and machine to insure coverage of area to be X-rayed. Mounts and labels X-rays.

—Maintains patient's record of treatment. Records oral conditions of the teeth and surrounding tissues, progress and therapy notes, appointments, and the number of patients treated and type of treatment administered.

Where to Start

A good starting point is your local library. Ask the desk librarian for a recent copy of *Federal Jobs Digest*. Reading it will give you a good handle on what's involved in working for Uncle Sam, plus there is a listing of national OPM announcements.

Contacting the Federal Job Information Center (FJIC) in your state (look under "U.S. Government" in the phone book) is another good move. The purpose of these centers is to provide general information on Federal employment, explain how to apply for specific jobs and supply application materials. You can get information by mail, telephone or by visiting a center.

In addition to the FJICs, you can call or write the chief dental officer of a VA hospital, Department of the Army, Navy or Air Force military installation. Ask if they employ RDHs at that facility, and, if so, do they anticipate any job openings in the near future. What you don't want to do is send them your résumé just on the chance there might be an opening. They don't file applications for unadvertised positions.

Federal Prisons

Depending on Federal budgets, opportunities for RDHs open up from time to time in Federal prisons. Although these correctional institutions are under the Department of Justice, each institution hires contract personnel according to its individual budgets, many of which allow for a permanent full-time or permanent part-time RDH. If so, the job is usually advertised in a local newspaper and snapped up quickly.

To get the jump on any job openings, contact the chief dental officer of an individual prison to ask that your name be kept on file in the event a position becomes available. (Unlike other Federal agencies, these facilities do hold résumés.)

Federal prisons, VA hospitals and military bases are listed under "US Government" in the phone book.

References

Office of Personnel Management, *Position-Classification Standard for Dental Hygiene Series GS-682*, TS-61, March 1982.

Dreyer Thomas, personal conversation with staff member of the OPM's Office of Standards Development, Medical and Legal Division, June 10, 1991.

RDH in Research

RDH in Industrial Research

Christine Hovliaras, *a clinical research scientist for a major manufacturer of oral health products, explains how a curious mind, determination and a keen interest can lead to success.*

How I Began My Journey

I think one of the most difficult things in life that a person must decide upon is "what do I want to be and how will I make a contribution to society?"

Like other teenagers, I thought of becoming many things. Then an event changed my life when I was 14 years old. I needed orthodontic treatment.

My orthodontist was an intelligent, authoritative, humorous man who impressed me with his vast knowledge of dentistry and his neurotic and endless passion for a healthy, clean mouth. After viewing a picture on the doctor's operatory wall, I was definitely motivated to keep my bands plaque-free. The photograph showed the mouths of two people: one person practiced excellent oral hygiene; the other did not. As you can well imagine, the sight of plaque accumulation and decalcification was enough to motivate me to floss and brush my teeth and gums on a daily basis! That was it. I would become a dental hygienist.

A Lucky Break

During the summer of my first year in the dental hygiene program, my mother encouraged me to seek a position as a part-time dental assistant so that I could gain experience in the routine operation of a dental office. Her reasoning was sound. I found a job as a part-time dental assistant in a busy two-dentist practice.

Fate has a funny way of affecting a person's life. In this case, it was fate and timing that I would meet a wonderful periodontist in this practice. Dr. Jeffrey M. Gordon has become my great friend, mentor and colleague. What a coincidence—and how fortunate for me—that he worked in the periodontics department and oral health research center at the same dental school I was attending for hygiene. My interest in research was beginning to take its first steps.

At this time, Jeff was starting a part-time periodontal practice and was looking for a part-time dental assistant. Of course I wanted the

36

job. The only catch was, I had absolutely no periodontal assisting experience. I put my inhibitions aside and approached him about the position. I explained that I wanted to learn this facet of dentistry and that I would be leaving this present job at the end of the summer. I remember telling him he wouldn't be sorry if he gave me the chance. That was eight years ago. I'm still working with Jeff one evening a week and enjoying it as much as I did when I started!

The Seeds are Being Planted

Jeff trained me to assist in all periodontal procedures: frenectomies, gingivectomies, gingival grafts, gingival flap and osseous surgery . . . I loved it. I became his right-hand person; he became my friend and mentor. When I graduated with my associate's degree and got my license, I became Jeff's dental hygienist, periodontal assistant and office manager.

I was determined to pursue a bachelor's degree. Jeff was very supportive of this. When I was a senior, he offered me a part-time research position in the university's Oral Health Research Center. What did I have to lose? I had more to gain—and maybe I would really like it! The seeds were beginning to sprout.

I began working with Jeff on a long-term antibiotic study. He taught me to evaluate gingivitis and plaque and perform accurate and reproducible attachment level and probing depth measurements. As the saying goes, "practice makes perfect," and with hard work and patience, I became experienced as a clinical investigator. Aside from my clinical responsibilities, I was given sole control over the appointment schedule and clinical supply ordering.

The work was challenging and interesting. I enjoyed being with patients and dental colleagues in this capacity. Research was much more than I had ever imagined. I began to realize how large a part it plays in the fabric of our lives. It is the nucleus of our being. Without it, life would not be the same and opportunities would be limited.

Pursuing Another Interest Simultaneously

At the time I received my bachelor of science degree, research was not my only interest. Teaching was another. I became a part-time faculty member in the department of dental hygiene for two years, teaching freshman and sophomore students.

Teaching was a great challenge for me. I learned patience, perfection, comradery, and a true appreciation for our profession—especially the educators! I wanted to make a difference in each of my students' abilities, to bring out their best, and to encourage them to succeed in their career and their lives.

About this time my part-time position in research led to a full-time position as a research dental hygienist/clinical investigator. My experience and bachelor's degree qualified me for the position. I was very excited. Full benefits, development as a researcher, a competitive salary, and networking with corporate sponsors. I was a little apprehensive—the way everyone is when beginning a new venture. But I knew I could do it.

Which Direction to Take?

I now had to decide where my career would actually take me. I knew the research position was a wonderful area to be practicing as a dental hygienist, but would I be happy in the same capacity five years later? I enjoyed both teaching and private practice, but I didn't want to do either full time. I wanted to sample different fruits (opportunities) from the same tree (dental hygiene profession). So I did. I worked as a researcher, educator and clinician and decided to further my education. I was very interested in industry—good old corporate America. The career of a clinical monitor and a product manager interested me greatly. I knew that to get ahead in the business world you have to be marketable. I also knew that the path to marketability is a master's degree in business administration.

Getting Ready

I researched available MBA programs. The pharmaceutical studies program filled my needs. The program offered education in the core business courses while providing an intensive, 24 credits in the pharmaceutical industry. The combination of a solid dental hygiene education and an MBA in pharmaceutical studies was the perfect match for me.

I began graduate school while working both a full-time and a part-time job. It was an exhausting few years. However, my positive outlook and perseverance kept me focused. I knew in the long run the payback would be two-fold. It has proven to be the right decision.

Shortly before getting my degree, I was notified that the dental school and the Oral Health Research Center would be closing. I had been working at the Center for five years at this point. Although shocked at the news, I felt as if one door was closing and another one was opening. That open door was the corporate world and I was more than ready to walk through it.

Digging In

With MBA in hand and my expertise in clinical research, I interviewed with several companies and selected Warner-Lambert, manufacturers of *Listerine* and one of dental hygiene's staunchest supporters. I've been with them for over two years now as a Clinical Research Scientist in the Dental Affairs department in the Consumer Products Research and Development Division.

My responsibilities as a corporate scientist range from writing study protocols and research reports to monitoring clinical test sites. I handle consumer, sales force and professional inquiries on our oral hygiene product line. I assist associations with professional programs and interact with marketing groups and advertising agencies. I keep current by reading dental hygiene and other professional journals.

I truly enjoy the challenge of this position. Each day is different from the previous day. Project deadlines, clinical study timetables, meetings, training courses, catching planes, attending conventions, responding to product requests are all in a typical day. The people I meet are a highlight of my job, especially the exceptional dental hygienists I come into contact with during the year.

I am also active in professional organizations. I've been secretary of the New Jersey Dental Hygienists' Association Board of Trustees for two consecutive years, alternate delegate to ADHA annual session, and president of my school's dental hygiene alumni association. I've also presented numerous continuing education programs to hygiene students, faculty and practitioners. All these activities have not only added a balance to my career, they have heightened my visibility within our profession.

How to Begin a Career in Research

If what you've been reading appeals to you and you think research might be a career goal for you to consider, here are some guidelines to help you think it through.

1. A formal education is a must. The minimum of a bachelor's degree in dental hygiene with a research concentration, or a B.S. in a specific relevant area is required. Graduate level study is preferred, such as an M.S. in dental hygiene or a related discipline.

2. Attending courses on research topics can be very helpful. These courses could include research design and methodology, research critique, statistical methods/tests, or Food and Drug Administration regulations regarding proper implementation and conduct of clinical trials.

3. Consider volunteering in a hospital or dental school research setting until a position becomes available.

4. Become a member of your professional organization so you can keep abreast of the issues facing our profession, hear about opportunities, and collaborate with your colleagues.

5. Keep current. Read dental journals and magazines to educate yourself about new products and methodologies.

6. Network with your dental hygiene colleagues. Start a study group. Consult people who currently work in an area you may be interested in.

7. Be assertive and ask questions.

8. Organizational and interpersonal skills are a must. A positive attitude and being able to work on different projects at the same time and meet deadlines are extremely important.

Words of Advice

Our profession and that of dentists are two small worlds. People know people and word travels fast. Some of the best advice I can offer is never to burn your bridges. There may be a time in the future when you may need a favor or are looking for a certain opportunity and need a person's assistance. You will be a much smarter and happier person if you abide by this information.

Your career is what you make it. Don't let other people who are dissatisfied with themselves discourage you. You are in control of your destiny. I truly believe that what one puts one's mind to and aspires to, one will definitely achieve. Nothing worthwhile is ever easy, but hard work, patience, a positive outlook, a sense of humor and an appreciation of people are the keys to success. Good luck to you!

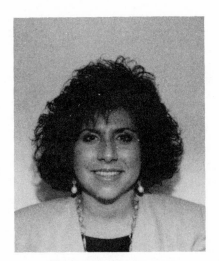

Christine Hovliaras

Working in the
Insurance Industry

Working in Dental Insurance

Cathleen Terhune Alty, *a professional writer and consultant, spent four years in medical and dental insurance in marketing, services, public relations and administration.*

When considering career options, dental hygienists and assistants often think about working in the dental insurance field. Based on their office experience, they believe that working in an insurance company means processing dental insurance forms. But there are many positions within the dental insurance industry besides claims that offer exciting career challenges.

How an Insurance Company Operates

To get a handle on how a typical insurance company operates, divide it into three parts: the claims division, which spends the money by mailing checks to dentists for work they have performed on patients; the marketing division, which brings in money by selling dental coverage to employer groups; and administration, which oversees and controls the marketing and claims divisions.

The claims department inputs data from submitted claim forms into a computer system for payment. Claims analysts review or "prescreen" claims to make sure the submitted forms are complete before they are entered into the computer. A verification department checks to make sure the data has been entered into the system correctly. If not, an adjuster corrects the error. Usually, dental claims supervisors manage the department after coming up through the ranks of processors.

To work in the claims department, fast and accurate typing skills are a must. Most insurance companies set quotas on how many claims each processor must enter per day as well as high accuracy standards. As many dental hygienists feel they are "people oriented" and want to use these skills, it is important realize that the claims department really has very little to do with people and a lot to do with paperwork, codes and fees. No degree is usually required for these positions. Salary ranges from minimum wage for data entry personnel to about $16,000 for lower supervisory positions.

Sales and Marketing

The marketing division is the true people-oriented department and the key to financial growth of the insurance company. Within this division there are marketing managers, sales representatives and many support staff positions. Marketing managers study the marketplace to target sales efforts and expected outcomes, make changes to benefit structures so they are more attractive to potential enrollees, and coordinate the efforts of the sales force and support staff.

Sales or account representatives are responsible for selling dental coverage to companies. Often sales positions are divided into two parts: new sales and renewal sales. New sales representatives bring in new companies and new enrollees, while renewal sales reps take care of companies currently covered by the insurance and make sure the employer group renews its contract with the insurance company.

Both positions require excellent communication skills and a commitment to service and unfailing persistence. The sales staff must fulfill sales goals or quotas. Usual 60 to 80 percent of their salary is fixed; the remainder is commission. Sales positions almost always include travel, entertaining clients on an expense account, and often irregular hours. College degrees are usually necessary for most marketing division positions, but this varies from company to company. Salary ranges for sales representatives, including commissions, are $25,000 to over $70,000, and $40,000 to $100,000 and beyond for upper level marketing management positions.

There are many marketing division support staff positions: enrollment, public relations, services and telemarketing. Assisting the marketing division through these support positions can be a good way to break into a higher sales or marketing position in the future.

Enrollment, PR and Services

The enrollment department assists the sales staff by mailing the booklet that explain coverage, maintaining data about new or existing enrollees in the computer. Salaries range from $13,000 to $25,000 for enrollment positions.

Public relations (PR) promotes the image of the company in the community and beyond. PR people may write the booklets and brochures used to explain coverage to new enrollees, handle promotions and advertising, hold press conferences or other media events, as well as create film or slide presentations for use by the sales representatives or company management. Salary range for the public relations manager, which normally requires a degree in public relations or journalism, is $35,000 to $48,000.

The services department usually has two parts: enrollee and professional services. Enrollee or customer service handles all written or telephoned questions and complaints from enrolled people. Professional services manages any problems dental offices may encounter.

Both positions require excellent communication skills, tact and patience. After working in a dental office, a person would no doubt have a lot of empathy for the people who call for help! Services can be a very rewarding area to work in and offers good chances for promotion throughout the company. Some insurance companies consider services duties under the public relations department or administration. Salary range is $13,000 to $25,000 and usually does not require a degree.

Telemarketing representatives usually screen all incoming sales inquiries and make "cold calls" to prospective clients. They turn over any leads to the regular sales staff and often share the commission if a sale is made.

Administration

The smooth, efficient and profitable operation of the insurance company rests on the administrative management team. These are by far the most challenging, as well as lucrative, positions in the company.

Managers determine policies for claims payment, approve marketing strategies, oversee investment of company profits, handle legal conflicts, plus a myriad of other responsibilities. Included in this division are finance and accounting, legal, management information services (computer programming and support), personnel, purchasing, and quality assurance/utilization review (to make sure dentists aren't billing for procedures they haven't performed, for example). All the upper management positions for claims processing and marketing are also found here.

Most of these positions require a specific degree but some of the support positions do not require degrees. The rising spiral of health care costs have squeezed insurance company profits to the limit, and the struggle to improve cost efficiency continues. New innovations are needed and the people who can meet the challenges will be greatly rewarded—but it won't be easy.

Seeing Yourself

If you want to work in a dental insurance company, you many see your dental background as a real plus. Unfortunately, the insurance company probably won't because they are largely unaware of what experiences you have gained in a dental office.

Communicating your experiences in terms a potential employer can understand (experience in sales, communication, organization, purchasing, public relations, etc.) will help as well as having determination to get the job.

If you are serious about wanting to work for an insurance company, willing to work in an entry level or assistant-type position and "learn" your way up, it won't be too difficult to obtain a job. Don't be discouraged if you are told the company is not hiring. Many insurance positions have a high turnover rate, and jobs are often created quickly to fulfill an immediate need.

Some dental insurance companies are divisions of huge medical insurance companies. As medical insurance premiums are higher than dental, there is more money to hire staff and often more positions are available. It may be wise to start in medical and then move to dental as those positions become available. Some companies combine medical and dental operations and staff work in both areas simultaneously.

Pros and Cons

Unlike most dental offices, you can expect a complete benefit package: full medical and dental coverage, life and disability insurance, sick and vacation leave, maternity/paternity benefits, retirement programs, and employee stock ownership plan, continuing education reimbursement, and other great benefits.

Work hours are standard except for some marketing division personnel and for part-time or second shift data entry personnel. If you have a small wardrobe, you may find it necessary to add appropriate business attire as it will become important to dress for the job you want to move up to (without overdressing your boss, of course!).

Working a 40-hour week can be an adjustment if that isn't your present schedule. Another adjustment can be dealing with the political atmosphere. It may be helpful to quickly learn the company's organizational chart to know who reports to whom and how information flows through the company.

The insurance industry can offer personal and financial growth, tremendous challenge and relative stability to your career. Having creativity, imagination, enthusiasm and a positive attitude can practically guarantee a successful career in dental insurance.

RDH in Dental Education

RDH in Dental Education

Cynthia Fong recounts her entry into teaching dental students. She is a past recipient of the Warner-Lambert/ADHA Award for Excellence in Dental Hygiene.

An Unplanned Beginning

A career in dental education was not a goal of mine when I entered the dental hygiene profession. In fact, one might say that I "evolved" into my current position. Despite my unplanned beginnings, I've found that being a dental educator is one the most rewarding career choices I could have made. Over the last decade and a half, dental education has provided me with opportunities not found in dental hygiene education, clinical practice or private industry. It has enabled me to grow both professionally and personally. Indeed, it is a career that I would encourage hygienists to consider as an alternative to traditional dental hygiene.

Gaining Credibility

Even while in hygiene school, I preferred providing oral hygiene instruction to my patients rather than prophylaxis services. I believe it enabled the patient and me to interact with one another. My preference probably explains why I was one of the first students to volunteer to take part in an extramural program to provide patient education to small group audiences at local area health fairs.

A month before I graduated, I learned that the dental school intended to employ a part-time staff hygienist to administer and coordinate the patient education program that I had volunteered for as a student. I applied for and obtained the position. Along with employment in private practice, I felt I had the best of both worlds.

As time passed, I began to look for new professional challenges. I realized that opportunities in clinical practice were limited and that any hope of advancing my position at the dental school would be unattainable because I did not possess an advanced degree. So, I returned to school in the evenings to complete a bachelor of science degree in business administration. I chose this major because it would give me the education and managerial skills necessary for advancement at the dental school and for employment in private industry.

Moving Ahead

As I was completing my bachelor's degree, the health fair program I had been working on was discontinued. Since I was pursuing a degree, I was reassigned to coordinate a newly established prevention clinic. The purpose of this clinic was to have a specific place for undergraduate dental students to provide their patients with preventive services such as patient education, prophylaxis, sealants, nutritional counseling, etc. (These services are identical to those provided by dental hygiene students but are termed "preventive dentistry" services when rendered by dental students.)

By the time I completed my degree, the prevention clinic was in full operation. I was again looking for new professional challenges. I could see my focus shifting toward dental education. As a staff RDH I could not assume any formal responsibility to teaching dental students. Yet I made myself available for questions concerning prevention and offered helpful suggestions to improve the quality of care provided.

The more involved I became with this aspect of the program, the more I loved what I was doing. However, I did experience some frustrations which resulted from my lack of a faculty appointment. Unfortunately, I could not pursue such an appointment until I had a graduate degree! So, off to school I went once again as a part-time student to get a master of science degree in dental hygiene education and administration.

Obtaining a Faculty Appointment

When I acquired my master's degree, I applied for a faculty appointment. The dental school had never before appointed a hygienist to its faculty, so a precedence would be set if it did so now. My application brought varied reactions from the faculty, administration and dental community, ranging from full support to the raising of questions about the legality of appointing a hygienist. Although deliberations continued for over a year, I was finally appointed to faculty as a clinical assistant professor.

I believe a critical factor in my success to acquire faculty status lies in the support I had of several faculty members at the dental school. Their respect for me as a professional grew over the decade I worked with them as a staff RDH. I developed their respect through my professionalism and concerted efforts to maintain open lines of communication with each of them. I'd share information with them about the clinical and non-clinical contributions a hygienist can make in the delivery of dental health care.

Currently, as a faculty member in the department of pediatric dentistry and community health, I am responsible for providing clinical and didactic instruction in preventive dentistry to undergraduate dental students through lectures, small group seminars and pre-clinical rotations. Throughout their junior and senior years, students render preventive care to their patients in the prevention clinic under my instruction.

Other Opportunities

In addition to my teaching responsibilities, I have the opportunity to conduct research, serve on school-wide committees and provide community service. Although a faculty member is not mandated to do these activities, promotion and advancement depend upon the extent of one's participation. Time is allocated during school hours to pursue scholarly activities for professional development.

The dental school also provides faculty with the opportunity to maintain their clinical skills by participating in intramural faculty practice. The environment simulates private practice and I perform clinical hygiene procedures here. For my services, I am paid an hourly salary in addition to my base salary.

Why I Like Dental Education

I thoroughly enjoy the challenges that dental education has to offer. Although I have the experience and credentials to seek a faculty position in dental hygiene education, I choose to remain in dental education because I believe that in my current position, I can better contribute toward building positive relationships between the two professions than if I became a hygiene educator.

My decision to continue to teach in a dental school is not all altruistic. The salary and benefits I receive as a dental educator compare favorably with salaries offered to dental hygiene educators and private practice hygienists. As I am promoted through the ranks and achieve tenure, my salary will increase proportionately.

My salary also takes into consideration the time I spend in non-school hours doing activities such as preparing and organizing for lectures and clinic, reading professional journals, attending departmental and school meetings. The fringe benefits far exceed those received in private practice but are comparable to those received by other faculty in an educational institution.

I believe my future in dental education depends solely on my own initiative. If I choose to continue to teach effectively, conduct research, publish extensively and actively participate in community service, I will have sufficient documentation to support an application for promotion and tenure. I also believe that if I were to complete a doctoral degree, it would expedite my advancement.

Although there are far more advantages than disadvantages to being a dental educator, there is one disadvantage I find quite disturbing: there aren't many hygienists who are currently dental educators.

In 1986, I conducted a survey to determine the number of RDHs who were employed as dental educators ["Employment of Dental Hygienists as Dental Educators," *Journal of Dental Education*, 1987:51 (10):597]. The study revealed that only a handful of hygienists throughout the United States hold faculty appointments in dental schools. As a result, I find myself with very little opportunity to interact or network with colleagues who are in the same position as I am. There is also a lack of dental hygiene/dental educator mentors who I can view as role models and utilize as resources. I believe that as more hygienists enter dental education, these problems will be eliminated.

What it Takes

If you want to pursue a career in dental education, you must possess an advanced degree. A minimum of a master's degree (a doctorate is better) would make your entry easier. Previous teaching experience would also be a plus.

Once your degrees and experience are in place, I suggest you explore the possibility of teaching in areas such as preventive dentistry, periodontics, community health, pediatric dentistry, geriatric dentistry or behavioral science.

When you begin seeking a faculty appointment in a dental school, expect competition not only from your dental hygiene colleagues, but from dentists who may want to enter dental education or be transferring from another educational institution. Don't let this deter you. Even though a dentist has the educational credentials to teach, an RDH has the advantage. The primary focus of our education is prevention oriented and hygienists almost always have a dedicated and enthusiastic philosophy toward disease prevention and health promotion.

If you are unsuccessful in obtaining a paid faculty position, consider volunteering your time as a clinical instructor in an appropriate clinic at a dental school. Even if you devote only a few hours a week, it will enable you to gain valuable experience and create mechanisms to network with existing faculty. Keep in mind that although it will not be easy, once you accomplish your goal it will be one you'll never regret.

I certainly wish you all the luck in the world.

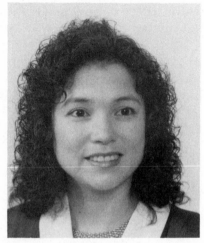

Cynthia Fong

Beyond Licensure: The Value of Continuing Your Education

Isn't an Associate's Degree Enough?

A question that frequently comes up is, "Do I need a bachelor's or a master's degree to get ahead in hygiene?"

The answer to that lies in what your goals are. Most clinical positions in private practice do not demand other than a license and the necessary schooling that goes with it. If, however, a practice or clinic structure offers senior positions or administrative responsibilities for an RDH, formally-acquired skills in supervising, training and management will boost the candidate into the senior slot.

Positions in alternative practice settings, public health, research, sales and marketing and other options outside of private practice frequently require a bachelor's degree. Given the demands of present-day certificate programs, many RDHs are close to completing their academic requirements for a bachelor's degree by the time they graduate. It may pay for them to finish their degree while still in that mode.

How To Do It

If you are already licensed, seek credit for your specialized training by building on what you already have, especially if opportunities outside the private practice environment are being considered.

Resources at many local colleges nationwide have expanded to recognize and give credit for dental hygiene training and background. At a time when traditional college enrollment is dropping, non-traditional programs are springing up to meet the demand for alternative approaches to learning.

The attraction of non-traditional eduction lies in the flexibility to receiving credits for a variety of learning experiences; credits by examination; credits for life experiences, independent study, correspondence courses . . . even computer networking!

These experiences are considered "external" in that the learning is obtained outside the traditional classroom setting. Instead of being institution-oriented, the non-traditional system is learner-oriented.

One hygienist who acquired her B.S. degree through an accredited external degree program after many years in practice, says, "In addition to wanting to move away from straight clinical hygiene into management, I also got my degree for personal satisfaction. My self-esteem shot upward. I now had confirmation of my knowledge and skills."

Finding out about degree-completion programs whether on-site or through a "university without walls" can be accomplished by researching what your local educational institutions offer and through specialized publications.

The American Association of Dental Schools has compiled a listing of degree completion programs nationwide. (Several are identified in the "Resources" section in the back of this book.) Orders for the publication, *Degree Completion Programs for Dental Hygiene*, should be addressed to Publications Assistant, AADS, 1625 Mass. Ave., NW, Washington, DC 20036. The price is $10.00 per copy (includes first-class postage).

Campus-Free College Degrees by Marcie Thorson addresses non-traditional learning. This guide to accredited off-campus college degree programs nationwide is a must for RDHs seeking an accredited bachelor's or master's degree while remaining at home, on the job, or geographically unable to go to a college or university offering an accredited program. Check with your librarian, the clerk in the bookstore, or call 918/622–2811 for ordering and pricing information.

Another useful book is Susan Simosko's, *Earn College Credit for What You Know*. This guide provides instructions for assembling and documenting a learning portfolio. Included is a resource list of colleges nationwide which participate in programs that recognize and award college credit for knowledge and experience. The cost of the book is $9.95 plus $2.50 for shipping and handling and can be ordered from the Council for Adult and Experiential Learning (CAEL), 223 W. Jackson, Ste. 510, Chicago, IL 60606.

Knowing What You Want First

According to Richard Nelson Bolles, the guru of career counselors, there are five reasons why most people want to go back to school.

1. They want to acquire more knowledge about a subject for intellectual rather than vocational reasons.

2. They want to pick up additional marketable skills to help them advance in their present field.

3. They want to acquire the requisite skills to change fields.

4. They want to stretch their mental capacity by undertaking an intellectually rigorous course of study.

5. They want relief from the world of work (otherwise known as the "perpetual student syndrome").

Which reason or combination of reasons applies to you?

Many times RDHs become professional students. That is, they take courses endlessly in the hope of finding a clue as to which career direction they should pursue. The reason why the task is endless is that they are going about it in reverse. Additional schooling is the means to the *objective*. If there is no objective, the means continue in a non-directed fashion and never really assume a shape.

Clarify your thinking as to what you want. Then find out if more schooling will bring you to fulfilling that dream. If you know what you want before you embark on your educational journey, you will not be disappointed in the outcome.

How Valuable is Continuing Education?

Hear the words of the 12th century physician-educator, Moses Maimonides. He said, "May there never develop in me the notion that my education is complete, but give me the strength and leisure and zeal continually to enlarge my knowledge."

Surely in that thought rests the nerve center of true learning: the love of inquiry for its own sake. Couple this with the professional pride and responsibility to maintain and increase one's skills, knowledge and abilities, and therein you have the philosophical base for educational development. One must keep growing intellectually or take a back seat to progress.

Sometimes, though, the feeling that we "know enough" creeps in, especially after completing years of arduous training and finding that our skills are not being fully utilized. Stamp that feeling out before it destroys your self-esteem. How much better to get respect and admiration from your patients who *expect* you to keep up, who *expect* to see your operatory wall covered with information on degrees awarded, licenses obtained, and continuing education courses attended. The image you create enhances your standing in their eyes, makes you feel better about yourself because you're actively demonstrating your interest in "keeping up." Continuous learning is one of the hallmarks of a professional, especially one who's licensed and needs to keep his or her skills on the cutting edge of change.

Many believe mandatory continuing education creates accountability on the part of the professional. The public often views this mandate as a kind of guarantee. It sends out a signal that there's a competent, educated person at the other end of the instrument, one who's up-to-date professionally.

Evaluating CE Courses

How do you know if the program you want is worth your time and money and is the right level for you? Course provider Marsha Raff Mayer claims there are five key points for RDHs to consider before committing time and money to a program. (This same information applies to both home-study courses and those on site.)

1. *Reputation of the sponsor.* If previous courses you've attended by this sponsor have been well-run and the speakers were dynamic and relevant, chances are this was the result of good, thorough preparation. You can expect to see the same qualities in action again.

2. *Relevancy to your job.* Does it sound as if there are some tips or new information that will be of immediate value to you in your work? If you are in doubt, call the sponsor and delve a bit into course content to see if it meets your needs.

3. *Hot new topic?* Does it appear that this particular topic hasn't been around before? Perhaps it is controversial. This may be your only chance to hear the information.

4. *Tried and true program?* Poor programs and speakers tend to develop a reputation for low quality and fall by the wayside. A program that comes back time and again must be pleasing its audiences. The bugs and weak spots have been worked out.

5. *Examine your own reasons.* If you only sign up for this course because you need the credits, the fee is low or the location is convenient, you will be courting dissatisfaction. The *subject* should be the deciding factor.

Keep in mind that your expectations may exceed what any one course can deliver. Not every course is going to be new material from start to finish. Go with the attitude that if, when you leave, the course has held your interest, built upon your present knowledge and offered some new information, your time and money were well spent.

Networking with Peers

Course attendance is a perfect opportunity to mix and mingle with your colleagues, find out who's doing what and where, reunite with former school chums and co-workers, and discover how you, your job and your career mesh with the total dental health care picture. You might even hear about new opportunities for employment.

Many benefits are gained from continuing your education through course attendance. You'll have the chance to keep abreast of the state of your art; gain new knowledge; exchange ideas and expertise with your peers and speakers; develop new skills; identify resource people; be energized and recharged; and expand your network of contacts.

You grow through continuous learning. As Dr. G. V. Black, one of the founding fathers of dentistry said, "The professional man (woman) has no right to be other than a continuous student."

RDH in a Hospital

RDH in a Hospital

Tom McGivern discusses his personal and professional growth in hospital dental care programs.

My beginnings in dental hygiene were a little unusual. First of all, I was the only male in an all-female class. More importantly, I entered hygiene school right from being a combat medic in Vietnam. Quite a change, but probably the reason why I've centered my career on serving the medically compromised.

My Philosophy

Like many of my classmates, I entered private practice right after graduation. After a few years, though, I knew I didn't want to say in this treatment environment. Although I enjoyed the work and had no problems with either employers or patients, I felt there was more to hygiene than being a money-making entity for a dentist. I wanted to make a difference in the lives of patients who really needed my care and dental direction.

One issue I had not been able to resolve in the private practice environment was that care was often rendered based on the patient's ability to pay. For example, instead of having the patient return for another session or two of treatment, I was often instructed to finish in one visit. This created an ethical conflict for me of what was in the best interest of patients when services were not covered by insurance or their ability to pay. I began to seek employment in an environment where I could practice dental hygiene without the bottom line.

This philosophy brought me to the National Foundation for the Handicapped, a non-profit organization operating nationwide. I learned of it though a dentist in my Army Reserve unit.

After a series of interviews and competition with other qualified candidates, I was selected to coordinate the mobile dental van program. My responsibility was to coordinate a schedule for specific schools and adult training workshops with the school nurse or hygienist in charge of the participating programs.

Our patient population was unable to seek dental care either because of their economic status and/or their handicap. So, we brought dentistry to them. I drove the van, setup the equipment, exposed and developed radiographs, and assisted the dentist during operative treatment. I really enjoyed what I was doing and decided then and there to continue my career "rooting for the underdog."

From that situation I moved into a hygiene position at a large medical center. Although most of my work was of a clinical nature, I had the chance to participate in the prenatal program. I'd meet with new, expectant mothers and discuss prenatal dental care, such as how to avoid tetracycline stains during pregnancy and after birth, and how to prevent nursing bottle caries in their baby. It was a very interesting job.

It was while I was at this center I responded to an ad for a dental clinic coordinator/clinical dental hygienist in a hospital dedicated to HIV-infected patients. I didn't know that much about AIDS at the time, but I knew I wanted to be a a part of this new era in dentistry resulting from the epidemic.

When I accepted the position, my family and friends were concerned about my proximity to the AIDS virus. After calming their apprehensions, I began work at The Spellman Centre in St. Clare's Hospital in New York City, a facility dedicated to HIV-infected patients.

Working at this center for HIV-related disease has put me in the forefront of dentistry. The challenge is still facing us ten years into this disease. This opportunity has been one of the best career moves I could have made and most rewarding both personally and professionally. I've met some of the brightest and most dedicated individuals it has been my pleasure to know in my life.

What the Work Entails

My job is hard and demanding. This disease has its cost in life, suffering to the patient and emotional and physical drain on the staff. But I believe that if you can relieve a person's discomfort and restore a better self-image, it is worth the effort.

Many of our patients feel a tremendous stigma resulting from their illness. We try to treat them as individuals with dignity and compassion. It is hard on us to adjust to our patients' mood swings and anger which result from medication and the loss of their friends. It's hard on us when our patients die. We do bond with some patients. In the nearly five years I've been here, I treat the patients with the assumption they're going to live a long life. When a patient crosses that patient-turned-friend line, I feel extremely sad when that person dies. Still, knowing I have improved the quality of life when it was needed most is what makes it all worthwhile and helps me get through this stage.

At the hospital, we have a multi-disciplined approach to the patient, incorporating dentistry, medicine, psychiatry and patient advocacy. Specialists range from social workers to case managers.

Our patients are on a three-month hygiene recall as the disease makes them prone to rapid periodontal breakdown. We evaluate any opportunistic oral manifestations such as candidiasis, apthous ulcers and Kaposi's Sarcoma (KS) and effect treatment accordingly.

Professional Growth

The move to the Spellman Centre has brought me advancement and opportunities as a dental hygienist beyond my wildest dreams. I lecture to dental and dental hygiene associations, at major dental meetings and AIDS training centers on oral manifestations of HIV infection and developing a practical infection control protocol in the office. I've co-authored abstracts which have been presented to international conferences on AIDS and an article which was published in the *Journal of American Periodontology.* I've been the subject of newspaper and dental hygiene publications. I've met with the presidential commission on AIDS and have been in contact with various world-reknowned health care professionals. Even though I knew there would be some media contact when I took the job, I am still amazed each time it happens.

Advantages and Disadvantages

My particular job notwithstanding, let me share with you what I feel are some of the advantages and disadvantages of practicing in a hospital environment.

ADVANTAGES:

1. Job security. One of the reasons I chose to practice in a hospital setting was to make up for the insecurity found in the private dental office. I have known RDHs who've worked for a dentist for ten or more years who were dismissed because they have reached the highest pay level they could, or because of personality or professional conflicts.

For me, job security is very important. As a male in a predominantly female occupation, I feel my position is less secure than my female counterpart. And I am the traditional breadwinner.

I feel that in a hospital I have more rights to grievance if I feel that a situation or working condition is not up to standards. In the hospital I'm in now, I had to join the Health Workers' Union. This does not mean I can't be dismissed, but the reasons would have to do with infractions of hospital policies. I feel more secure with this form of mediation.

2. Opportunity for self-improvement and education. There are countless lectures provided on site in disciplines other than dentistry. At a teaching hospital, when residents receive seminars on new techniques and theories, I can attend. There is always a wealth of information available.

3. Great benefits. As a union member, I belong to a panel program which provides comprehensive medical care for me and my family at no cost. I have the option to go outside the panel which means the plan would pay a percentage and I would pay the difference. I'm also covered by disability benefits should I be unable to work due to a medical condition. In private practice, the inability to work results in no pay and possible loss of the position.

4. Social interaction is outstanding. We have social activities such as interdepartmental softball, boat rides, employee recognition parties and of course a Christmas party. These activities allow us to talk and have fun and to recognize our co-workers as individuals.

DISADVANTAGES:

1. As a condition of employment, you may be required to join a union. Some people feel this diminishes their negotiating power. They may not agree with the union philosophy or the contract negotiated with the hospital.

2. There is always the possibility of being a "number" in the hospital bureaucracy. This can result in feeling a loss of individuality.

3. A hospital is a very stressful work environment. More often than not, most hospital dental patients cannot access dental care for a variety of reasons, some of which are related to a poor dental attitude. In treating such patients, you can experience a "why bother?" attitude yourself. If you do, you will burn out quickly and create problems for yourself both on the job and at home.

I have shared with you my story about working as a clinical hygienist in a hospital environment. I hope my experiences will in some way be of help to you in your future endeavors in dental hygiene.

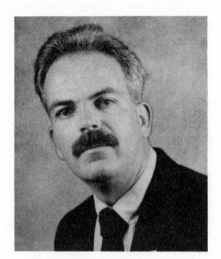

Tom McGivern

RDHs in Private Practice

Coordinating a Soft Tissue Management Program

Mary Roper Hurley *tells of her upward mobility in private practice.*

When I graduated from dental hygiene school over twenty years ago, I was filled with excitement about working in private practice. I couldn't wait to get out into the real world and start plugging in all that I had learned and practiced in school. But the real world of the dental hygienist in private practice turned out to be, for me, a downward spiral of monotony, time constraints and physical demands. For many of my colleagues, though, private practice was a dream come true. The big question was whether or not I could make hygiene more exciting, challenging and fulfilling for myself.

Meeting the Challenge

On numerous occasions I tried to change my frame of mind through different approaches to private practice. When psyching myself up every day to not let the "beat the clock" routine get to me didn't work, I asked for more time per patient. When that wasn't granted, I divided my time among general practice, ortho lab work and teaching settings. This maneuver provided a welcome variety in hygiene duties and made the hectic pace of general practice not seem inundating. Being in teaching also gave me the opportunity to see a need for more and better media for teaching dental hygiene and medical subjects. I decided I wanted to try that and went off to graduate school 3,000 miles away to study mass communications.

All through graduate school I found myself needing to work in private practice both because my economic status demanded income and because I missed it! I worked in a perio office first. Although I learned a tremendous amount there and experienced a whole different dimension of hygiene, I found myself slowly gravitating back to general practice.

I then worked in a couple of general practices while I produced and successfully marketed media for dental hygiene. I really enjoyed writing and producing media programs. To be able additionally to sell them and instruct teachers in their use was icing on the cake. I thought this type of job might be one I'd like better than hygiene. But the vast amounts of personal and professional time needed to be committed to these endeavors, and the small amount of financial return, were significant drawbacks I needed to deal with.

The way I handled this situation was getting a job as a communications specialist at a major medical X-ray company back east. During my five years in this position, I honed my writing skills, acquired hands-on experience with videotape production, and learned about the art of printing. Even with all this stimulation and fulfillment, I still found myself working some Saturdays in hygiene, just to keep my hand in and just because I missed it.

Shifting Goals

When corporate politics started to overwhelm me, I decided to return to private practice part time and see what I could do incorporating my communications experience with my hygiene skills. My goal was to do some hands-on hygiene and use my skills as a writer to develop materials that are so integral a part of all dental offices.

The doctors in the private practice in which I settled were open to hearing about my past frustrations with hygiene scheduling and eager to plug in the skills I had to offer as a hygienist and a writer. Both the doctors and I wanted to develop a framework that would help us provide the level of treatment each patient required at each recall. As it stood, the schedule was set up on the assumption that every patient needed the same amount of time to have maintenance needs met.

After trying various approaches, one of the doctors found a home study program that contained all the basics necessary to get us headed in the direction we wanted to go quickly and easily. The program was not a new concept nor did it propose novel treatment modalities. It was simply soft tissue management easily placed in the capable hands of the hygienist. The program calls for the hygienist (or dentist) to assess a patient's current level of oral health, propose appropriate treatment, make judgements, motivate patients, use refined levels of scaling and root planing, and determine subsequent appointment times.

Building Team Support

Our whole office was pretty revved up about the program. The hygienists were excited about the potential it offered them to have variety in their schedules and to use more of their skills. The doctors were thrilled that the hygienists felt so positive. The front desk staff was initially concerned and somewhat resistant. However, once they became more familiar with the additional insurance codes and treatment plans that we would use, they, too, got on the bandwagon about the program.

Getting started was easy. We listened to the home study program and extracted the pieces we wanted. Then we designed new pieces we felt were necessary and/or worked better for us than those that were provided. For example, we produced a package of written materials about the program for promotion and patient information. This process was especially fun for me because I got to write the materials and handle the production of all the package pieces.

When that step was completed, we used a team approach for the rest of the preparations. The doctors and staff worked together to prepare standardized insurance forms for all possible treatment plans in the program. (These forms would allow quick, easy paperwork in the treatment rooms and at the front desk.) We also designed our own plaque and bleeding record and our treatment record. The assistants and hygienists worked together in figuring out tray setups, planning inventory control on oral hygiene aids and standardizing home care instructions. The front desk staff familiarized themselves with new, standardized insurance sheets, more codes and scheduling needs.

We then had a few role-playing sessions among staff to get familiar with presenting our program to patients, working with new records and fielding possible questions and problems that might arise.

Implementing the Program

It took a few months from the time we started talking about using this program until the time we actually used it with patients. That was in the spring of 1987. Exactly four years later, all maintenance patients in this practice have been evaluated in what we call our dental fitness program.

In this program appointment times for maintenance checkups are set according to the level of oral health patients present with at their last maintenance visit. If the screening exam (which is done prior to starting the preset treatment) indicates the need for additional or alternative treatment, the framework of the program streamlines the transition into it and the presentation of it to the patient.

All new patients in this office automatically receive the program's criteria during their initial visit (and this visit is with one of the doctors). But it is the hygienists who usually carry out the steps delineated in the soft tissue treatment plan.

What This Program Means to Me

This dental fitness program has changed my schedule from one of monotony and drudgery to one of diversity and challenge. Instead of prophy after prophy, I may have blocks of time for quad scales with anesthesia, perio scales, reevaluations and oral hygiene instruction sessions interspersed with the routine prophys. It makes all the difference in the world.

Another plus of this program is the high level of oral health of the patients in this office. Being a part of that accomplishment and knowing that I have helped create a solid foundation of sound perio health upon which the doctors can build gives me a great deal of fulfillment and personal satisfaction.

In addition to all the advantages of the program I've already mentioned, it has also helped me find my niche in hygiene. I now know that to keep myself recharged, I may need to leave a certain job, but I don't have to leave the profession. Rather, I can bring all my skills to hygiene, create a different job description and be instrumental in initiating and implementing new concepts.

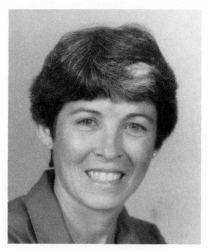

Mary Roper Hurley

Working With an Assistant

Laura Mallery-Sayre, *a past recipient of the Warner-Lambert/ADHA Award for Excellence in Dental Hygiene, traces her history of practicing creatively.*

A Solid Education

Creativity, along with diversified educational and employment opportunities have been the keys to my success and longevity in dental hygiene practice.

It began with a four-year program that allowed for critical thinking and applauded creativity. From the first day of classes we were treated as colleagues by both the dental hygiene and dental faculty. We were encouraged to work with the dental students on a referral basis and to follow our patient's progress through the various departments. Our opinions were sought on the patient's dental hygiene progress, but we were educated to think beyond the scope of dental hygiene practice to the total health of the patient. Functions that are still considered as expanded in some states today were routine education for us. We were trained to think ahead. This solid foundation was essential to my success as a professional.

The Beginning

No dental hygiene program truly prepares a student for the shock of entering practice. Learning the knowledge base and technical skills is just a drop in the bucket of what constitutes dental practice. Dental offices rarely operate under the same guidelines taught in school. I learned after my first job experience that if you want to practice in a certain type of environnment and are concerned about the overall care the patient receives, it is best to interview the dentist rather than the other way around. Once I got that straight, life got much easier.

The first office I worked in I had never seen. The dentist was on the faculty at the testing facility where I took my state boards. He hired me during the exam! It was quite a shock when I discovered there was no means of sterilizing instruments, no curettes (only sickle scalers), and the hygienists saw a patient every 30 minutes. The practice literally supported a periodontist.

I fought the dentist and other hygienists every day over values and cried myself to sleep every night. My view of myself as never being a quitter kept me in that practice for four months. I'd like to think I made a difference while I was there but I probably didn't. That practice, however, had a profound effect on me. I was very clear about not being willing to sacrifice my ideals and values for anyone.

The next dentist was virtually interrogated. He'd been trying to hire a hygienist for three years but his major drawback was that his dental hygiene operatory was a converted closet. However, he supported my ideals, purchased an autoclave and curettes, and gave me total control over my patients' appointment times and hygiene therapy. I was quite happy working in that closet for three years. I watched my patients get healthier and I felt continually rewarded. I saw eight patients a day, five and a half days a week and made very little money. But money was not the key issue for me; self-satisfaction was my driving force. It was this quest for continued growth that led me into teaching.

I taught in two universities in two very politically different states. One state had an enlightened state board of dentistry—here I taught expanded functions; the other was operating in the dark ages. The second school was taken to task for teaching functions that were outside that state's dental practice act. The school lost their legal battle (they believed they could teach under academic freedom) and I took it personally. I became politically active.

I campaigned to have a dental hygienist placed on that state board of dentistry and was successful. I testified before another state legislature to persuade them to eliminate preceptorship training for dental hygienists and was unsuccessful. I became a line officer for the component, state and national associations and chaired more committees than I wish to recount. My battle against the boxes had begun.

Breaking with Tradition

My return to clinical practice in 1975 marked the beginning of a new era in dental hygiene for me. I threw away my cap, set up two dental hygiene operatories and hired a full-time dental hygiene assistant. I overlapped my schedule and maximized my dental assistant to the full capacity of her training and legal barriers for practice. I saw as many as 16 patients a day (including children), increased my services and my quality of care to my patients and minimized my stress. My personal and professional growth soared. My income quadrupled. My ideals were still intact and I had broken through another traditional barrier. I told anyone who was willing to listen about it and even discussed it with a few who were not. Four of my assistants from this practice went on to become hygienists. It was great fun. We loved our patients, we did beautiful dental hygiene, and we were making a difference in our community.

Life Changes

In 1981, I was afforded the opportunity to be a member of the first dental hygiene delegation to China. That trip changed my life. I was asked to chair another delegation to China, and a dentist I met on the trip arranged for me to lecture in Hawaii. (That dentist later became my husband!)

Through my several visits to Hawaii to lecture and provide in-office management seminars, I realized what wonderful employment opportunities this state offered an RDH. The supply of dental hygienists was limited, the demand and need were high, and the dental community was fairly progressive. A dental hygienist was already serving on the Board of Examiners and there was legislative movement afoot to introduce local anesthesia and general supervision for dental hygienists. While these may simply appear to be political issues, the rules and regulations governing the practice of dental hygiene strongly affect a hygienist's ability to maximize his or her capabilities in providing care to the community served. It was a definite deciding factor for me. It was going to be difficult for me to leave the east coast. I had my home, my friends, my practice. I made my choice. I needed to move forward again, to continue to take risks.

I returned to school to complete my master's degree while working for an instrument manufacturer as their national program director. It was a rough time. I managed to live on three hours of sleep a night for the better part of a year. I had an office in my home, a full-time secretary and a WATS line. It was the most productive year of my life. I really got to know my strengths and weaknesses. I spent an entire year being petrified of failure and had none. I learned that my only limitations to success were those that were self-imposed.

Making the Move

I moved to the island of Hawaii the first part of 1984. I had to wait until April to take the national boards; July for the state exam. In the meantime, two dental offices needed an office manager and I split my time between the two.

Beginning anew is a humbling experience. In this instance, my educational background was really tested. It proved to be invaluable. Within eight months we had revamped the office scheduling, implemented accelerated hygiene practices within both offices, established production goals and increased collections. The next step was deciding where and how I wished to practice once my license came through.

Two offices were compatible with my philosophy of practice. Their dentistry was excellent and their patients were their number one priority. Both offices were interested in change and valued dental hygienists as colleagues. They were both willing to let me take charge of the dental hygiene program.

Now, telling someone with my history that she can take charge of *anything* can be dangerous! I remained controlled, however. The most damage I did was to hire two assistants instead of one for the accelerated practice. That's actually pretty radical considering the scope of dental hygiene practice nationwide.

How I Practice Now

I work two days a week in one office where my practice is limited to initial therapy on and maintenance of advanced periodontal patients. The other three days I work with my husband (which is another whole chapter) and again see mostly those patients who are advanced. Another dental hygienist works for us on the days I am not in the office and my dental hygiene assistants work with her.

Our assistants are cross-trained to work with either the dentist or the hygienists. Since nearly all are trained on the job, they start with me first. Sterile technique, infection control and patient management are presented before they sit chairside. Four-handed dental hygiene, radiographic technique and theory follow.

The assistants greet and seat the patients, update medical and dental histories and red-flag them. They take blood pressure readings, have the patients fill out a recall card, take any treatment-planned radiographs, disclose the patients, use non-directive counseling in reviewing oral hygiene instruction, fill in services rendered forms, assist the hygienist in charting head and neck findings on both soft and hard tissues, provide four-handed support during anesthesia, root planing or prophylaxis, and prepare the operatory for the next patient after the current patient is released. This includes the cleaning and sterilization of all instruments as well as tray setups for future patients. Meanwhile, the second assistant has seated the next patient and has gone through all the preliminary workup with them as the last patient is being completed and released.

It is a smooth operation, but it doesn't happen without a great deal of effort. Training and refinements are continuous. We have staff meetings and training sessions every week. We spend numerous hours with the entire staff at continuing education courses. Communication is the key to success in this type of practice and we have a personal counselor who works with us as individuals and as a group.

The staff have to be willing to change to allow for the continual growth of the practice. This factor is extremely important when selecting staff members. We practice team hiring. This means everyone gets to vote and everyone gets to support the new member.

We have a pension/profit-sharing plan for the entire staff as well as bonuses if we go over production goals. If a staff member is well all year, in addition to getting well pay, that person gets a two-day, all-expenses-paid trip for two to the Hawaiian island of his or her choice.

We provide uniforms, medical and dental coverage and continuing education coverage. We have a huge party every time one of us has a birthday, and we celebrate most of the minor events that come up as well. We want our staff to know that we value them not only as co-workers but as friends. We work hard but we have fun!

Keys to Establishing an Accelerated Dental Hygiene Practice

1. There must be a minimum of two operatories available for dental hygiene functions.

2. The dental hygienist works with one or two dental hygiene assistants and has the ultimate authority in the hiring, training and evaluation of such assistants.

3. The scheduling coordinator works directly with the dental hygienist in establishing guidelines for treatment scheduling. This coordinator has the responsibility for scheduling, confirming and receiving the patient.

4. The dental hygienist establishes the time frames needed for each type of service per each patient's individual need (gone are the days when everyone gets a flat 45-, 50- or 60-minute appointment).

5. The dentist and dental hygienist consult continually about patient treatment plans, progress and specialty referral. This is not a 9-to-5 program. It requires a lot of outside work and expands dental hygiene beyond a job and into the professional realm.

6. Continuing education for the dentist and dental hygienist is mandatory. State-of-the-art dentistry is a must.

7. The entire team needs to be involved in office goal-setting and must be committed to its achievement.

Working on Commission

My remuneration agreement is definitely a change from the norm. I work on a 40 percent commission. The dentist gets a 40 percent commission from my production, and 20 percent is used to pay for my assistants' salaries and my supplies. This year, my baseline production appears to be approximately $156,000. Since I do most of my lecturing and traveling in the first six months of the year, production is invariably higher at year end. My production is significantly influenced by the amount of root planing I do. This varies considerably from month to month. My first three years of practice in Hawaii were financially outrageous because I had such a huge volume of root planings. Since then, it has evened out and I have a larger maintenance practice to accommodate.

Summing Up

I have been privileged to wear many hats in dental hygiene: clinician, educator, lecturer, adminstrator, instrument designer, researcher, consumer advocate, change agent. For nearly 20 years I've been a political activist within ADHA, working for change to promote the art and science of what I believe is a true profession.

But it is as a clinician that I have found my highest rewards. As far-fetched as it may sound, every patient is a challenge for me, every root surface is a new educational experience. I mentally devise new ways to get around problem areas on nearly every periodontally-involved patient. I firmly believe that there is always a better mousetrap to be developed. I have never been satisfied in staying static with my skill level. My need for constant improvement has driven me crazy; my need for constant change has driven my staff crazy. After all these years, dental hygiene is still a challenge to me. And practicing creatively makes it *fun!*

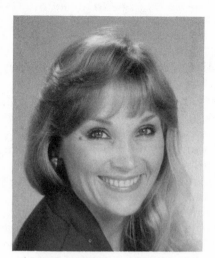

Laura Mallery-Sayre

Expanding into Cosmetic Dentistry

Lynn M. Miller *reviews the role of the RDH in this burgeoning dental specialty.*

This decade is a time of incredible excitement and challenging growth for dental hygienists wanting to expand into the cosmetic area of dentistry. The discipline is constantly changing as new materials and procedures are developed in tooth bleaching, bonding, veneers, inlays and crowns.

Cosmetic dentistry can enhance our roles and give us an entirely new perspective. By understanding smile design, we can open up new avenues for our patients to increase their self-aareness, offer them another view of how the world sees them, and provide ourselves with stimulating new opportunities.[1]

Our patients' perspective of dentistry has also changed. Because of the media, television and movie-star perfect smiles, the once conservative consumers who just wanted to be relieved of pain or have healthy mouths now have new expectations. Our patients are becoming more aware of how their smiles can improve their looks, their lifestyles and their work.[2]

Our educational and clinical background have not prepared us for these new challenges. We therapeutically treat and educate our patients based on the status of their current periodontal infection, or we help to eliminate or prevent carious lesions via the application of sealants. We are experts in disease prevention, but do we know what we can provide for our patients in the area of smile enhancement? Do we know how to evaluate face shapes or how the lips frame the smile. Do we know the elements of smile design? Do we truly understand how a person's life can be virtually transformed by a beautiful smile?

Since the basic science courses have been the foundation of our clinical skills, we can now build on them as well as utilize the psychology and human relations courses we took in school. We can express our sensitivity to and awareness of color and design. With this foundation, it is easy to understand cosmetic dentistry and how it applies to us professionally.

An Awakening

I will never forget the first day I was in a cosmetic dentistry practice. After working for six years for a periodontist, I thought I had mastered all the necessary clinical skills for any area of dentistry. I was wrong.

During our team meeting, the dentist asked me if I planned to use acidulated phosphate fluoride on my mid-morning patient who had porcelain veneers. Of course I was going to use APF; it was the best fluoride to remineralize enamel from thermocycling or enzymatic breakdown of food. He informed me that APF ruined porcelain. In fact, many cosmetic dentists use APF to etch porcelain before bonding another porcelain piece for repair. As for stannous fluoride, it releases a tin ion that can stain composites and the resin around a porcelain restoration. (For the patient with a high caries rate, recommend a sodium fluoride rinse for daily use.) All this was news to me.

From that day on, I started my research. I found that most of my rote routine in my operatory would ruin much of the new cosmetic restorations in my patients' mouths! I was appalled. I began asking my colleagues and dentists if they knew what patients needed or wanted from us before or after cosmetic restorations. No one knew.

Here patients were spending all this money to get gorgeous smiles with porcelain veneers, indirect and direct bonded veneers, indirect or direct composite restorations, crowns, inlays or onlays, and when they came back for their recall appointment, we hygienists were undoing what the dentist had so carefully done.

I learned a lot from my research. I also learned that the first step to changing my routine was to recognize differences in materials.

How to Identify Porcelain from Composite

Run your explorer over the surface of the restoration. All porcelain feels scratchy, like a china cup. It is the hardest restorative material in the mouth. Because of this hardness, porcelain can cause abrasiveness to the opposing dentition. Therefore, routinely polish porcelain on all occlusal and incisal edges so that any roughness caused by normal grinding or bruxing will be polished out.

When an explorer glides over a composite restoration, you'll feel a relative softness. There is no scratchy feel like that of porcelain or even enamel. There are two types of composite restorations: microfills and hybrids. Sometimes they are both used in a layered fashion for a more esthetic effect.

A microfill composite, normally placed in the anterior part of the mouth, is the shiniest type of composite. It has the advantage of being the least porous and the most stain resistant of all the composites. Because of its esthetic capabilities, it is more like enamel.

A hybrid composite is much more stress resistant than a microfill. It is used in posterior restorations most of the time, but if the patient has a crossbite, cuspid rise or end to end occlusion, it is sometimes placed in the anterior. The finish on a hybrid composite is not as shiny or lustrous as a microfill. Don't expect the same finish when polishing.

How to Polish Porcelain and Composite

Whether a composite is made in the lab as an indirect veneer, inlay or onlay or applied directly on the tooth in a one-step office procedure, microfills and hybrids are polished exactly the same. Aluminum oxide polishing paste is the only polishing paste made for these restorations. (All types of pumice-based polishing pastes will scratch composites.) Apply the paste directly on the tooth with a cotton swab, put a drop of water in your prophy cup and polish for 30 seconds.[3]

Porcelain veneers, inlays, onlays and crowns should be polished with a diamond polishing paste. This paste keeps the surface glaze smooth so that the restorations will not abrade the opposing dentition. The only time this paste is contraindicated is if composite resin is exposed. (Composite resins are used to cement these restorations. Diamond polishing paste can scratch and ditch composite resins.)[4] Shofu Dental Corporation has designed an "Esthetic Maintenance Kit" which has all the tools necessary to polish, remove stain and maintain these restorations.

The final step is to topically apply sodium fluoride for four minutes.

Planting Seeds for Smile Design

Smile design takes into account the shape, contour and symmetry of the lips and how the lips frame the teeth. To evaluate the symmetry of a smile, focus on the midline and allow the teeth to flow out to the commissure (or angles of the lip). The entire picture should be a uniform color. The centrals should typically be about 10 to 11mm in length and .5mm longer than the laterals. The cuspids should be about the same length as the centrals. This entire picture should be one of symmetry. There should not be one tooth that stands out because it is crooked, discolored, or shorter or longer than the others.

Look for a chip or overlap that interrupts this symmetry. Does it make us feel uncomfortable when we look at that person's smile? Now go back to the midline. Is the maxillary and mandibular midline in the same position? Is the midline in the same midline of the nose?

Is the shade of the teeth too yellow or gray? Is there color symmetry? Are there any diastemas? Do the size of the teeth relate to the patient's facial and body design?

Finally, a healthy smile line is one that follows the slight curve of the lower lip. Think of it as the arc of the teeth flowing with the curvature of the lip.

Even if your patients have been with you for a long time, look at their smiles as you have never looked at them before. Ask yourself how this person's smile can be improved. All too often we assume our patients of record are not interested in having their smiles improved. Or they were previously told that nothing could be done. For years dentists have been taught it was virtually malpractice to cut into a fundamentally healthy tooth. Obviously, this approach has changed but many of our patients still hold onto this school of thought. It is our job to help them discover the potential beauty in their smiles.

Our patients do not see us as gaining monetarily for wanting to improve their smiles. They see us more as a friend with a caring yet educated viewpoint. They appreciate and deserve our input.

Getting Started

1. Look at the major fashion magazines—both men's and women's. Notice the models' teeth. Occasionally you'll see a smile that breaks the rules but typically the models have healthy, symmetrical smiles. Study the teeth color, how the lips shape the smile, the smile's symmetry.

2. Notice how aging it is on your patients when the smile is straight across. Try to visualize how this same person would look with a healthy smile line.

3. Talk to your dentist about his concept of smile design. The concept is only now becoming universally understood.

4. Take into consideration the lips as they frame the teeth. Look at the gingivae. Are they healthy? Are the gingival contours of the teeth symmetrical? Apply the concepts we discussed earlier.

What Else You Can Do

When you see inflammation in the gingivae surrounding a composite or porcelain restoration, talk to your employer. He or she will appreciate your care, concern and taking the time to communicate about the procedures. Your patients will appreciate your expertise in keeping their investment both functional and esthetic for the longest amount of time possible.

Keep a daily journal of questions your patients have or you have which cannot be answered at this time. Commit the next year to finding the answers, to learning everything you can about the new world of cosmetic dentistry. By raising your level of knowledge, education and ability to plant seeds, you will be worth a million to your doctor, your patients and to yourself!

"We can have everything in life we want, if we just give enough other people what they want."

—Zig Ziglar

References

[1]Jenny, J. Proshek. Visibility and Prestige of Occupations and the Importance of Dental Appearance, Journal of the Canadian Dental Assoc., No. 12, 1986, pp. 987–989.

[2]Brothers, Joyce "Are True Attractions Only Skin Deep?", *The Houston Post*, December 1988.

[3]Miller, Lynn M. Maintaining Esthetic Restorations (Houston: Reality Publishing Co., 1989) p. 38–65.

[4]Ibid.

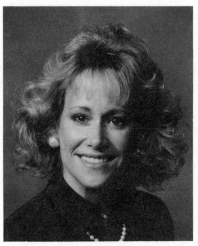

Lynn M. Miller

RDH as Office Manager

Donna Grzegorek *discusses her evolution from clinical dental hygiene to a management position within an orthodontic practice.*

In 1975, at the age of 15, I began working with a very progressive state-of-the-art orthodontist. My job description was varied but included basic administrative tasks, some clinical dental assisting, and elementary lab work such as pouring and trimming models. The doctor took great interest and time training me to a high degree of clinical competency.

Two summers later—still a part-time employee—I was performing tasks identical to those of the doctor's full-time chairside assistants. And at a comparable level of success and efficiency.

Noticing my enthusiasm for dentistry, the doctor put me in charge of his Personal Oral Hygiene (POH) program. This was a three-day program established to teach oral hygiene techniques and nutrition to our orthodontic patients. Being responsible for this program taught me so much. I knew I wanted to make a future in dentistry.

My Formal Education Begins

When I graduated high school, the doctor asked me to work full time in his wonderful office. I turned down the opportunity because I wanted to pursue a career as a dental hygienist. I was seeking a position in dentistry that would offer me more independence in my role with patients. However, I did work part time in this office while attending hygiene school, and maintained the oral hygiene program.

While in hygiene school, I developed an interest in speech patterns and sound reproductions. In search for more knowledge, I attended college as a speech pathology student, working as a clinical RDH part time. I came to realize that speech pathology was pulling me away from my chosen profession, dental hygiene. I elected to leave the program and recommit full time to my career as a dental hygienist.

Full-time Clinical Hygiene

When I returned to my community, I was again offered a full-time position in the orthodontic office. Very graciously, I declined. I

84

couldn't see where an ortho office would have need for an RDH. (Boy, was I wrong!) I sought employmnet as a traditional dental hygienist and secured a position in a very busy group practice.

At the end of the first year I was at my wit's end. I was bored. I felt stagnated. I was frustrated. Clinical hygiene was too routine for me. I was feeling very confused about my growing distaste for our profession. I knew I loved being in dental health. I loved working with people. I loved being in a position of knowledge and authority. I loved teaching and motivating people. But I was not happy. What was missing was the variety I needed in my workday.

I felt the need to speak with someone who knew me, who was familiar with my career objectives, who understood the role I wanted to play in dentistry. I met with my favorite orthodontist to discuss my current dissatisfaction. By the end of our meeting, I admitted I was ready for a change. The doctor asked for the third time to come back to his office full time as an "Orthodontic Hygienist." This time I accepted.

I must admit I was very skeptical about this change. I was still unable to see the numerous benefits a hygienist could bring to an orthodontic office. I was worried that my hygiene education would be wasted. But most of all, I didn't want to lose the independence being an RDH afforded me.

A Change in Attitude

A smarter move I could not have made. I learned that an orthodontic office can thrive with the knowledge and skills of a dental hygienist. I loved my new position! I found that every skill I had acquired in hygiene school and used in general practice was being utilized in this specialty practice. Indeed, I was not taking periapical or bitewing radiographs; I was taking cephalometric and panoramic radiographs. I utilized my polishing skills on each patient having brackets placed. I used my scaling skills on all patients post-bonding. I fulfilled my oral hygiene education and instruction teaching home care programs. My perio background came into play with our tissue management program.

The orthodontic cementation process is almost identical to sealant procedures. Most certainly I was teaching and motivating my patients in the area of orthodontic appliance maintenance. I was able to do periodontal evaluations for our adult patients and TMJ muscle examinations.

We implemented an orthodontic scaling program for our problem hygiene cases. Here I had the opportunity to work hand in hand with local periodontists to achieve positive results. As an orthodontic hygienist I was the natural choice to do treatment planning and consultation with the new patients and their parents.

During my phase as an orthodontic hygienist, I began to recognize the need for a better understanding of the orofacial musculature as it relates to skeletal form and function. My previous interest in speech pathology was modified to an area of study more closely related to dentistry. I pursued education, training and internship as a myofunctional therapist. I began to do myofunctional examinations and some therapy for our patients. I also incorporated a successful habit elimination program into my routine.

It should be obvious how much I loved the career change I made to an alternative practice setting. I met each day with many challenges and a never-ending amount of variety.

Another Opportunity

One year later when I thought I could not be happier, the doctor asked me to be office manager. Once again I was faced with a decision regarding my career. I was so happy with the current role I played chairside. However, becoming office manager was a promotion in my mind and an opportunity to gain knowledge in the business end of the practice. I accepted the position with some trepidation. I was again concerned about being pulled away from the clinical environment I had grown so accustomed to and that I loved so much.

This new job description had its own set of trials and tribulations. At this point I was 23 years old. I had worked with this office in many different capacities during the previous eight years. I was now cast into a job description that required me to delegate authority to people older than myself, to people who had once told *me* what to do. I learned very quickly that as a decision maker you were not and could not be everyone's friend.

My New Role

My new role involves interviewing, hiring, training and termination of employees. I am responsible for performance reviews, salary reviews, motivation, behavior modification, staff meetings, payroll, accounts payable and receivables. Trouble shooting and problem resolution are always part of my day.

I introduce new products into our office regime, film video t₁
tapes, develop training manuals and examinations. As th
hygienist currently in the office, I am responsible for certain c
procedures, particularly myofunctional and perio examinations
muscle exams and maintenance of our orthodontic scaling prog

My most recent exploration as office manager has been mark
both internally and externally, as well as some advertising. I
enjoy doing consultations involving treatment planning and final
arrangements for our new patients. And, since I have worn every
in this office at one time or another over my 16-year history, I am
prime candidate to fill in when someone is absent or ill. I enjoy
"break" in my routine to be receptionist, lab tech or chairside as:
tant for a day.

The variety in my job is endless. I am very happy with the directi
my career has taken. I'll always have traditional clinical hygiene
fall back on should I need it. In the meantime, however, I am deve
oping my skills in the areas of personal relations, management, bus
ness, accounting and marketing.

The current dental hygiene salary in my area (outside Chicago
ranges from $19–22 per hour. My annual salary is within that range
along with benefits including three week' paid vacation a year, holi-
day pay and sick days.

I've supplemented my formal education with continuing education
seminars and courses in marketing, advertising, personnel management, business practice, and of course, dentistry and dental hygiene.
I stay very active in my local hygiene component and state association. Both are excellent resources for learning.

I firmly believe education is the key to success. I make it a point to
learn something new each day. It can be a piece of knowledge big or
small. It doesn't matter what it is as long as your eyes are open for the
learning opportunity. After 16 years in the same office, I am proud to
say I am still learning something new every day.

Why Office Management?

A dental hygienist is the perfect choice for the position of office
manager. He or she has a higher degree of formal education which
places the individual in a position of respect among office peers. The
hygienist's commitment and dedication to dental health, the experience in personal relations, the detail that is demanded in the hygiene
curriculum . . . each of these prepares the hygienist to be meticulous
in management and organization. Hence, successful in the role.

A very dear friend of mine once said to me, "For every door that closes, two open up." I say to you, don't close your eyes; look for that opportunity. It's out there. As dental hygienists we have the knowledge, skill and expertise to wear many hats. If you are inclined to try another hat, do it! You might be as pleasantly surprised as I was.

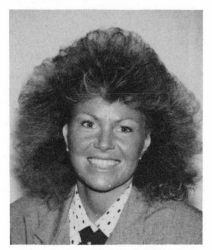

Donna Grzegorek

As Educational Resources Administrator

Linda Hirce Martin *tells how she successfully reshaped her job more than once in the same practice.*

You may wonder what the functions of an educational resources administrator are. I'll try to give a brief history of what has taken place to facilitate the need to create this position.

I've been involved as an RDH with the same periodontal specialty office for the past 18 years. Contrary to what you might think, it hasn't been the same job, day after day and mouth after mouth. The periodontist heading this office is progressive in his approach to dentistry, highly motivated, quality oriented, and most of all, sincere with his employees as well as patients, family and friends. If it weren't for his ability to allow staff to reach for their highest level of competency, I would still be in those 8mm pockets, complaining about everything around me and not seeing the light shining off polished enamel.

How it Started

My first responsibility in this office was as a full-time clinical hygienist. After about ten years, I began to suffer from Carpal Tunnel Syndrome and had to lessen my patient load. The office needed a full-time RDH, not one who was part time and in questionable health. I had some decisions to make.

My concern was in finding a replacement who would be willing and able to take on the added responsibilities I had assumed over the years. That was unrealistic. And I wasn't able to just turn my back on the patients and staff. Also, it would have been difficult (if not impossible) to find another office of the same high caliber even if the idea of leaving had entered my plans. How could I be productive without compromising my arm function?

I spoke with my boss about the possibility of using my knowledge in another capacity. He saw the benefits of a long-term employee functioning in another role. We discussed different ideas and came up with one of clinical staff supervisor.

Staff had always been receptive to my teaching new methods or offering ideas. I liked doing it. They had also been comfortable sharing problems and ideas with me instead of bringing them to the doctor. So it was a natural progression to change my duties from full-time hygiene to staff coordinator/educator—with some hygiene on the side.

A New Opportunity

It's been eight years since we made that first transformation. The job description has fluctuated with the demands of the office and staff. We've now come to another transitional point in the development of the practice, and again I am changing with the situation.

Our office has grown over the past years, not only in size but in knowledge. We now have two full-time periodontist/implantologists, a full complement of clinical and administrative personnel, and a very active 15-member study club. The last is what really tripped us into another dimension of professional interaction.

With all the internal growth of the practice coupled with the desire to become a resource center for the referring office network, the need for a coordinator to pull together the goals of the study club was imperative. I took over the task of becoming the educational resources adminstrator, a job still continuing to evolve by trial and error and as diverse as the name implies.

The science of implantology has opened up opportunities for every dental staff member. The entire staff of an implantologist must be educated in what implants are, why they benefit patients, and why it is imperative to be a strong, supporting team for the referring doctors. We became the nerve center of this development.

In our office we are learning about the patients' need for implants, how to answer their questions, and how to help them make financial arrangements. Every member has become involved, not only the clinical staff. We've found we have to include our referring dentists and their staffs in the learning and coordinating process. This way the lines of communication are two-way and we all know what we are doing.

Our Objective

The main objective of our new movement was to establish a study club that allows offices of diverse specialties to interact in the management of the partially edentulous patient. What this means is that a group of dentists are willing to share their ideas and their talents to formulate treatment plans for difficult implant cases. Every member of the group benefits from the learning experience. And pretty soon each member's staff will, too. We hope to expand the study group format to include clinical and administrative staff members in the near future.

My boss and I work together in setting up the study group meetings and try to provide the group with a variety of informative topics. While setting up these topics, I've become aware of the vast amount of resources there are for inter-office training. I pass this information on to the study group members for their staff, and also keep records for future inquiries. One of my responsibilities is being available to other offices' staff members for any training or assistance they may desire. This is in keeping with the idea of becoming a resource center for our referring dental community.

While we are finding it is important to have lectures, of greater value is the challenge of having a patient with a problem sitting right there and the group discussing various methods of treatment. This has worked beautifully and is a learning experience we all enjoy. I coordinate the patient with the meeting time and the dentist presenting the case and arrange for study model casts, X-rays and other pertinent material to be duplicated for the members. During the meeting, I function as a clinical assistant, recording secretary and business administrator.

Benefits to Me

The educational aspect of the position—such as expanding the implant knowledge for myself and staff—is the most rewarding to me. But please don't misunderstand. My position doesn't just revolve around implants. It happens that this is the direction of our growth at this time. I'm sure that as we become more familiar with all the aspects of this science, our focus will expand to incorporate other new and exciting dimensions of dentistry.

I am learning that what pertains to our office may also be applicable and important to our referring offices. I've had to stop thinking in terms of *my* office. With the specialization of dentistry today, one can no longer work in a closed dental environment. All the professionals must interact to benefit the patient. This is the best way to provide comprehensive care.

Reaching Further

Perhaps you're thinking this kind of position could only exist in a periodontal or oral surgery specialty because of the number of dental offices which need to be involved. I'm not sure those are the only situations in which it could work.

There could be a way of approaching several dentists and becoming an educational resource for them as a group. Or perhaps your employer already belongs to a study club. See what those members think of the idea. You would need to become familiar with the office policies, the methods of treatment and what is expected from staff. From that point, you would be "on call" to train the staff as they were hired or moved to another position in the practice.

If your employer wanted to expand on a treatment method, for instance, you would be the one to find the most time-efficient, cost-efficient and most clinically correct method. At that point, other staff members would be trained by you under the guidelines established by the dentist.

When I think of all the ways the dental referring community can interact, I don't know if I'll have time to do it all. But I'm trying! And you can, too.

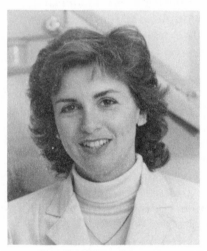

Linda Hirce Martin

In Veterinary Dentistry

Marsha Venner *explains how her dream of becoming a veterinarian was fulfilled by combining two disciplines.*

After working full time in clinical practice for three years after graduation, I could feel myself becoming burned out. I decided I wanted to pursue my dream of becoming a veterinarian.

As an interim to this goal, I became certified as a veterinary nurse. Then a lucky thing happened where I could combine my two licenses and degree. I became involved in a very new field in veterinary medicine called veterinary dentistry. This all came to be at The Veterinary Hospital of the University of Pennsylvania where a veterinary dental program was just starting up. I was in the right place at the right time.

Starting Out

I first started working part time at the hospital and part time at a human dental practice. As time went on, I got more involved with the research aspect of the program as well as clinically with the veterinary students. I progressed to four days a week at the veterinary hospital and one day a week at a dental practice.

I was so excited about my new job! There was constant mental stimulation as well as improving my self being. That is, I got involved with research, writing and public speaking—all the things I never in a million years thought I was capable of doing.

The dental service was combined with a head and neck surgery service. Students and an intern and surgery resident rotated through on a two-week rotation. My week consisted of one day in clinics seeing clients with their pets. At the end of the day, the group would have rounds with the students to discuss the case and set up the treatment plan for the animal. It was during these rounds that I learned about pathological diseases of the head and neck.

I soon discovered that veterinary dentistry was almost similar to human dentistry. I also discovered that I had to keep up with my knowledge of dentistry because the students were constantly asking questions. My second day was spent in surgery with the students, clinically teaching them the use of curettes and how to perform a proper dental prophylaxis.

As time went on, we realized very little research was being done on veterinary dentistry. To become more credible in the field, we began quite a few research projects. So, my third and fourth days were devoted to research.

As I became more confident in my knowledge of this specialty, I began giving continuing education courses as well as "wet labs" in veterinary dentistry. Most of my lectures were about periodontal disease in dogs and cats, the dental prophylaxis, extractions, care of dental instruments, and dental radiology. Publishing in veterinary nursing journals and of my research projects soon followed. Through my speaking engagements, I was able to travel throughout the United States and overseas.

The Rewards

It all sounds so glamorous but the truth is my salary was cut in half from being a full-time human RDH. However, I was willing to take that cut and supplemented my income by working as a human dental hygienist one day a week. The tradeoff was the constant mental stimulation, the excitement of a new field, the meeting of new people, and nothing was routine. I was extremely happy. It was worth it.

When an animal has a mouth problem, you know it. Very often they stop eating, mope around, and there is some sort of halitosis. I'd take care of the problem and there'd be a whole new animal. The owner appreciates this. That's very rewarding to me. I also get excited seeing students gain knowledge through my instruction. I also feel good about advancing veterinary dentistry through my research.

What I Do Now

In 1990 I decided I wanted a change from living in the northeast, so I took a job in a private referral veterinary dental practice in Houston, Texas. Of course it is very different from academia. Since it is a referral practice only, we have to educate the local veterinary community on the need for dentistry. There is a lack of veterinary dental education from the veterinary schools themselves. This means that vets are very unaware of dental problems. We make up for that lack.

A lot of marketing goes into running this practice. For example, we pick a particular dental problem and send newsletters to the local veterinarians.

Now that I'm in private practice, I'm more involved with total patient care than I was at the hospital. My duties in the practice are taking a medical history, getting preoperative blood work, putting the animal under anesthesia, doing dental prophys, root planing and curettage, taking radiographs, charting, performing minor extractions, assisting in more advanced dental procedures, and discussing home care with the client. You can see that a background in veterinary nursing is needed.

The salary ranges from $13.00 to $15.00 an hour; my day begins at 8 AM and ends at 5 PM. I am still very involved with speaking to veterinarians and their technicians.

My Goal

My goal is to become involved with academics two days a week and private veterinary dental practice three days a week. I enjoy teaching and learning—which is what I get out of academia, and I enjoy my clinical work—which is what I get out of private practice.

If you are interested in pursuing a similar path because of your love of animals, I'd suggest you go to your local veterinarians. Tell them what you're doing. Ask if there's some way to work together. Even if you begin by sharpening instruments you'll be serving a real purpose. You can then take it from there.

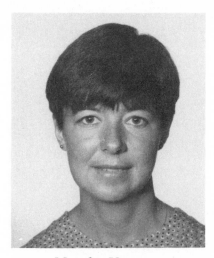

Marsha Venner

Ethical Development
in Dental Hygiene

Ethical Development in Dental Hygiene

Phebe Blitz *has a rich background as clinician, educator, administrator and consultant. She actively promotes philosophies and techniques for delivering the highest standards in quality patient care.*

When I first started in dental hygiene, "ethics" seemed a simple issue of "right and wrong," "shoulds and shouldn'ts." I had been raised in the midwest, and my sense of right and wrong was black and white. Gray was not a familiar color!

My early days in dentistry reflected those beliefs and my ethics were determined by what was "right." This was usually defined as "putting the patient first."

When I began to practice dental hygiene, I wanted to be sure my quality was the best it could be, so I always worked hard to please the dentist and make sure he was satisfied with the quality of my work. After I left that practice, I soon found another dentist who discovered my 30-minute prophys were not as high quality as I had thought. This became my first lesson in "ethics from within."

I had based my ethics and definition of quality on a source outside myself: laws, morality of society, association ethics, and, in this case, the judgement and evaluation of another professional. It was comfortable to rely on all those sources; I didn't have to take responsibility other than to follow the dictates of authority. It was much the same as I had unquestionably followed the dictates and authority of the law, society's morality and my parents when I was growing up.

Twenty years later, I can see the issues more clearly. My values have evolved from a list of rules from an outside source to an internal integrity that demonstrates respect for each individual and that person's opinions and beliefs.

I believe that any decision I make must support the self-esteem of everyone involved, including myself. I also believe I need to be clear in communicating my beliefs and open in listening to the beliefs of others. In growing into these beliefs, I have gained tremendously in self-esteem. I have come to realize that what I do in the office does make a difference. I take responsibility for my actions.

What Ethics Is

Webster defines ethics as the morality of a profession. Philosophers through the ages have argued from many points of view. The Greek philosopher Aristotle viewed ethics as a value to be strived for, one that is the basis of harmony in life and personal happiness.

Many religions adopt a set of standards defining moral or ethical behavior. Dentistry and dental hygiene have adopted a set of standards, a code of ethics, which defines the ethical behavior of the practitioner of that profession. Humanists, on the other hand, tend to view ethical behavior as being responsible choices a person makes in relation to the community and self. This would imply an internal set of standards or values used by the professional in decison making. It might also imply that the values could change as responses to choices are evaluated.

In general, societies have laws as required codes of behavior. Professions have codes of ethics as requirements for behavior, and individuals have values as bases for behavior. When any of these—law, ethics or values are not in agreement in a situation—there's stress on the individual. It becomes an energy drain causing fatigue and burn out.

Likewise, when people working together have different ethics or different values, they will make different decisions on the same issue. The lack of alignment of values among team mates can cause severe stress on each of the team members.

Analyzing the Problem

My second confrontation with an ethical dilemma came several years after the first. I had just joined a new dental practice. The interview process had gone well. Both the dentist and the staff seemed to be caring, quality conscious people. There was a new office, new instruments, and a one-hour time schedule for my patients. I was delighted! For the first few months I was so busy familiarizing myself with the office procedures, the patient personalities and the gingival and periodontal status of the patients, I didn't notice the consistency of open margins and recurrent decay.

As time went on, it became clear that poor dentistry was contributing to the need for more dentistry which was contributing to the breakdown of health and early loss of teeth in many patients. It became clear that the effects of my dental hygiene work was being compromised by the dentistry being done. It was also clear that my definition of quality was very different from the dentist's. In fact, his definition conflicted with my ethics which insisted on providing the best quality service for all patients. Still looking at ethics from a simple right and wrong paradigm, I chose to leave the practice.

This decision took me out of an ethical conflict situation and certainly reduced my frustration. It did not, however, solve the problem for the doctor, staff or patients. From my vantage point, 20 years later, it was an unethical solution to an ethical dilemma. An ethical solution is a win/win option where dentist, staff, patient and hygienist all benefit from the solution. Put another way, I had robbed a moment of opportunity from all the team members in order to reduce my own frustration.

Interestingly, I got another chance at this one. I soon found myself in a similar situation, a practice that I really liked for a lot of reasons, but the quality of dentistry was again in question. I didn't want to make another change in employment, yet I wanted my patients to have the very best quality of service. The options I could see at this time were:

1. I could leave as I did before. This would reduce my frustration. It would not help the patients.

2. I could stay and let the situation be. This would fulfill my ethical responsibility to the dentist, but it would not fill my responsibility to the patients.

3. I could discuss the problem with the dentist. This could result in getting me fired. It could also be a learning experience for the dentist and myself. I knew this solution would be difficult for me to do as I did not like conversations with authority figures.

I thought back to my previous situation with my very first job when I thought I was doing such quality dental hygiene. I remembered the dentist who let me know that my quality needed improvement. I was not pleased to hear that message and yet it had become a turning point in my career and, in fact, in my personal development. Had he chosen to fire me and find a better replacement, I might never have had a chance to improve my quality. He had provided me with that moment of opportunity and I took it. I knew then I needed to discuss the problem with the dentist.

The result proved to be a learning experience for the dentist and for me. At first he was not pleased to hear what I had to say; in fact, I thought I might lose my job. But I was careful in my conversation not to judge his work. My goal was only to provide facts from patients we were both familiar with and show concern over their dental health. I shared my ethics and values as they related to the patients. It turned out to be a very positive discussion. He became aware of some quality deficiencies. He looked more objectively at his work and began to find other things that needed improvement. He began taking continuing education course. We began to discuss team quality assurance at staff meetings. I didn't lose my job.

Contemporary Ethical Dilemmas

The issue of HIV-infected patients has brought many legal and ethical issues to the forefront. Recently, I heard a dentist say he had fired a dental hygienist because she refused to treat an HIV-infected patient. There had been quite a confrontation in the office. The result was an ultimatum: treat the patient or lose your job. The hygienist left the job with no discussion.

Now, the action of the dentist is consistent with legal requirements not to abandon patients. It is also consistent with the ADHA's Code of Ethics which requires hygienists to "serve all patients without discrimination." It shows respect for the patient—but it shows no respect for the fears or beliefs of the hygienist. In fact, the hygienist was concerned about the welfare of all the other patients as she knew the infection prevention procedures in the office were not adequate. If as much concern had been shown for the staff as for the patients and communication was valued, this situation might have had a happy ending for everyone involved. Again, a moment of opportunity was missed!

Another Example

A friend of mine came home from work last week suffering the stress of an ethical decision, although she didn't call it that. She was just frustrated and tired over a situation she had at the office.

Mr. Jones had appeared at 8 AM for his appointment with her at the periodontal office where she was employed. Her schedule allowed an hour. The procedure to be done was listed in the chart as scale and root plane the upper right quadrant.

After greeting the patient and reviewing the medical history, she started in. As she worked on the upper right first molar, she experienced difficulty in two ways. First, the pocket seemed deeper than what was noted on the chart. Second, there was an obstacle in the way. It looked like a tooth-colored filling. She assumed it must be a temporary since it was not flush with the tooth and seemed to be a "blob" in the way.

She struggled with the instrumentation in the deep pocket and around the filling and wondered what she was really supposed to be doing. Obviously, the area could not be definitively completed in the time scheduled. She continued and told herself to do the best she could under the circumstances.

She was still frustrated when we saw each other that evening. She indicated that her frustration was from not knowing what was expected of her by the dentist. I perceive her frustration to be from making an ethical decision to follow the instructions of her employer (as indicated on the chart and on the schedule) when it conflicted with her values and ethical responsibility to provide the highest quality of care for the patients.

Again, good communication could have solved the problem. Clarifying probe scores, expectations and the nature and purpose of the filling material would have provided an opportunity to learn for both the dentist and the hygienist. Consensus would have provided better quality care for the patient.

Where to Start

How can hygienists develop in this sensitive area? First, you have to know your own values. There are many values inventories and exercises that will help you become aware of and clarify your values. Study the ADHA's Code of Ethics and see where it is consistent with your own values. Are there any conflicts?

Find out if your office has a set of values or ethics. A mission statement or a patient's bill of rights might give you some insight into the values of the office. This is usually done as part of a team meeting or retreat.

The first step is having the individual team members define and clarify their own values. Then they come together to discuss different values styles and discuss the influence of each of these styles on the decisions that are made in the office. Now staff can formulate a code of ethics using the common values of the team members.

Once this is done, align the personal values of each team member with the code of ethics of the office. This is a clarifying activity that can help solve future problems before they arise. After you are satisfied with the office code of ethics, make it available to patients. Frame it and put it on the wall. Include it in the next billing. Hand it to patients as they come in for their maintenance appointments. Put it in a newsletter. Ask the patients for feedback. It will stimulate their thoughts on ethics, too.

It's always better when making an ethical decision to talk over the issues and possible solutions with another person. A different perspective can enlarge understanding of the problem and often find solutions one person hadn't seen.

The hygienist can also act as a facilitator in using the group process to solve ethical dilemmas. He or she can help the team work through the process so everyone can learn and be involved.

Your career in hygiene is full of ethical decisions. Some are clear cut and easy; some are difficult and stressful. All can be a challenging opportunity for growth. Helping the office develop in this area can be a new and important role for you.

When RDHs Become Disabled

RDH and Disability

Teryl Moyer *turns a physical disability into an income-producing career as consultant, writer and lecturer.*

Adhesive capsulitis. Frozen shoulder, they called it. It really didn't matter. Ready or not, I had just received a knockout blow from one of the many unique physical maladies which all too often ring the final bell for a clinical dental hygienist.

"I'm sorry, but it looks like your career is over." The doctor's somber prognosis left me stunned. The physical pain was nothing when compared to the months of emotional agony which followed. The depth of my panic soon revealed that a great deal of my self-esteem and personal identity had revolved around an image of being a caring and competent professional. That image was being erased.

Now divorced and suddenly careerless, without any alternative training, significant cash reserve or disability insurance benefits to sustain me, my life was on the ropes. Amidst the endless bouts of physical therapy and heavyweight dosages of anti-inflammatory medications, I was also faced with the seemingly insurmountable task of "patching together" something coherent from the shredded remnants of a twenty-year hygiene career.

During the following few weeks, a lot more than my shoulder was frozen. My mind dove into an icy, self-pitying, angry, frightened, despondent paralysis; quite contrary to my natural style of being an incorrigible, upbeat go-getter. I worried, and fretted, and cried, and slept, only to begin the downward spiral again upon awakening. I felt just like my arm, refusing to move in any direction more than an inch or two. I was undeniably "stuck."

Getting Unstuck

They say we never really know what we're made of until we're tested. My *test* had actually begun almost a month before, but so far, I was failing miserably. That eventual realization made me angrier than ever, but this time my anger proved constructive, releasing the energy and creativity I needed to finally detonate this dangerously myopic, self-defeating mind block. Treasured old adages began to rise from the rubble and boot me in the backside. Who said Life is fair? If

Life were fair, they'd call it *fair* . . . but instead, they call it Life. The *purpose* of Life is to discover your gifts and talents; the *meaning* of Life is to give your gifts and talents back to the world. When Life brings you lemons, Teryl, get busy and make some lemonade!

So, rather than recount an ever-growing list of liabilities and limitations, I decided instead to squeeze the lemons for a brand new list of personal abilities and assets. The process started slowly, but as one idea fed another, page after page soon filled with an astonishing tally of vastly diverse talents and fascinating options, all silent dividends from what had always before seemed to be a rather simple, straightforward career in dental hygiene.

No doubt about it. I could take these talents *anywhere*. But did I really want to give up a career in dentistry? It was time to make a choice.

If I want to stay with my current practice, I speculated, why not shift from the operatory to the front office? I already know all the patients, all the personnel, all the practice philosophies, policies and procedures. I could have those office management systems down in nothing flat!

On the other hand, I could just as easily move into sales with any number of dental products manufacturers. I certainly know the market inside out and backwards. In fact, come to think of it, I'd be great in sales of any kind . . . as long as I believed in the product. After all, that's really what I've been doing all along anyway, isn't it? Selling health to people? I've been moderately successful even under the least favorable circumstances, when patients are emotionally apprehensive and physically uncomfortable. Surely I could sell something to someone when they were relaxed and genuinely interested.

Hey, what about communications, or marketing, or public relations? That sounds like fun! I've dealt with a new personality every hour for more than twenty years. I'm not exactly a newcomer when it comes to establishing instant rapport with a lot of different people.

Then again, I might make a crackerjack dental hygiene instructor, or a hygiene program administrator. Maybe I should refocus my career toward public health or dental research. Why not public speaking or freelance writing? I have some great ideas, and someone might just want to hear them!

Suddenly my mind was ablaze with endless possibilities. I'd never felt so animated and alive! All my options seemed exciting, even the ones outside of dentistry. But I kept coming back to the one I still cared about most: fighting and *winning* the battle against periodontal disease.

A Bold Beginning

I scrambled to the phone and boldly announced to a long-term attorney/friend, "I want to be president!" I borrowed a few thousand start-up dollars from my family and hired the best marketing, financial and legal advisors around. Within weeks, I was CEO and OEO (only executive officer) of the fledgling corporation, Intercept, Inc.

I didn't have a clue how to run a business, but I had a clear vision of what I wanted to create and enough blind enthusiasm to fuel a rocketship to Mars. I remember my accountant shaking his head quite a lot those first 18 months. "This really shouldn't have worked," he'd mutter, "but somehow it did."

I knew why things were working, but somehow it didn't seem appropriate to share the little piece of personal philosophy that was guiding me so flawlessly through these most precarious of times. You see, I've always found that total naïveté, when properly applied, can be a marvelous attribute. When we don't know what's possible, many times we can do *im*possible things.

My goal was to create an unsurpassed "one-stop, in-office" consulting service where dental professionals could quickly access all the latest information on conservative periodontal management. Top quality all the way. No compromises.

It had taken me more than three years to gather, research, learn, and fine tune all the technical and behavioral data which had eventually revolutionized the way I treated my own periodontal patients. I knew, from my own clinical experience, that periodontal disease could be stopped dead in its tracks more than 80 percent of the time, *without surgery*, when treated like the bacterial infection that it is. I also knew that all these techniques, when artfully taught, could be learned in just three days' time!

My shoulder might keep me from actually *practicing* this technique, but it couldn't keep me from *teaching* it to other progressive professionals who wanted the best. If I could share what I had learned, rather than helping a few patients a day with my own two hands, I could potentially help thousands! That prospect blew my mind.

It still does. Because in these four short years, that once faraway dream conceived in the mind of a desperate, displaced hygienist, has grown into a vivid reality. Five extraordinarily dedicated and talented dental hygiene consultants are now stretching their professional horizons by carrying the Intercept message to progressive practitioners across the United States and Canada. We're making a difference, a BIG difference. And that difference has made an enormous difference in each and every one of us.

A Blessing in Disguise

Do I miss my career in clinical hygiene? You bet! I miss the smiles of my favorite patients, the challenge of a difficult case, the result that surpasses even my loftiest expectations. I miss the security of a steady paycheck, the luxury of closing the door behind myself at week's end and totally forgetting about work until the rooster crows on Monday morning. But would I trade what I've lost for what I've gained?

Change is never easy. Most of us go kicking and screaming into our Life transits, only to one day discover that the terrible crisis we encountered was really a blessing in disguise. Mine certainly was. It caused me to reach inside and find the courage to shift my focus and to make that leap of faith.

Without a frozen shoulder, I might never have discovered the joys of teaching, of setting my own schedule, of doing things exactly the way I think they should be done. I doubt I would have conversed with many of the giants of our profesion, or overcome my fear of public speaking, or written the books or enjoyed the financial abundance which now occasionally nets more in a single month than I have ever made in an entire year of chairside practice. I question whether I would have witnessed the splendor of New England, or fished the flats of the Florida Keys, or hiked the majestic Rockies above Calgary without this work that finally takes me there.

Perhaps a frozen shoulder, carpal tunnel syndrome or a bad back isn't the end of the world for RDHs so afflicted. Perhaps it's just the beginning. And maybe it's true . . . maybe we never really do know what we're made of until we're tested.

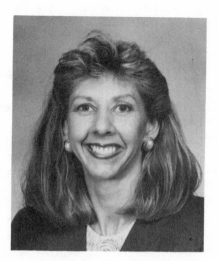

Teryl Moyer

RDH in a Dual Career

RDH in a Dual Career

Mary Y. Holston *describes how her interest in total patient care led to merging dental hygiene with nursing.*

Even as a child I knew I would become involved in the world of dentistry. My mother was a certified dental assistant and worked with her brother, a general dentist. Together they taught that one's smile showing good healthy teeth made an attractive greeting.

When talk of careers came up in conversation, my mother would encourage me to consider becoming a dental hygienist. Her closest friend was a hygienist working in the same office. She earned in a three-day week what my mother earned in five and one-half days. She easily convinced me that dental hygiene offered time to enjoy the income made while working in a profession that was exciting, interesting and challenging. And so I pursued a bachelor's degree in dental hygiene.

Making a Decision

After practicing in the private sector for one year, I accepted a teaching position with the same school I graduated from. For several years I enjoyed teaching both didactic and clinical courses to first- and second-year dental hygiene students. Rewarding as it was, I felt an inner desire to know more about the whole patient and the interaction that the oral cavity had with the other body systems and vice versa.

After giving this desire a great deal of thought, I reached the conclusion that I didn't want to abandon the dental hygiene profession altogether, but wanted to expand and incorporate its possibilities within the field of medicine. To remain in dental hygiene and become a part of the medical team meant I had to find territory which combined the two fields. Oral and maxillofacial surgery offered what I considered the best potential meld of the two disciplines.

Taking Action

I spoke with the chair of the university's department of oral and maxillofacial surgery. He listened to me with interest and enthusiasm. I then moved to that department and began developing dental hygiene within its parameters.

112

About this time several surgeons became involved with orthognathic surgery. I began actively working with them in this area and witnessed how the interaction of orthodontics, psychiatry, speech pathology, periodontics and surgery affected their patients' projected surgical outcomes.

My own responsibilities included obtaining clinical records, i.e., radiographs, models, tracing the projected cephalometric radiograph, and obtaining preoperative photographs for all scheduled orthognathic surgery patients. When the patient was ready to go to surgery, I was responsible for coordinating the records and seeing that everything was in the operating room on the morning of surgery.

At first I could do little in the OR but watch while standing on a stool behind the working surgeon. But this was an important and valuable period, since I absorbed the techniques of each osteotomy and was able to continue figuring out how, as a hygienist, I might become even more involved.

My active OR participation began as an assistant scrub nurse. This person remains "sterile" throughout the entire surgical procedure and is responsible for instrumentation and watching the sterile technique of the participants. This assignment enabled me to learn the instruments and anticipate the surgeon's needs as the procedure progressed.

The Interest Grows

My interest continued to grow as I witnessed other nurses, interns and residents perform procedures important to the team effort in accomplishing the surgical goal of both patient and surgeon. It wasn't long before I recognized that a huge gap existed between the medical and dental teams.

The nurses had no idea why a dental hygienist was present—or even wanted to be. Some were annoyed, some inquisitive, others apathetic. I noticed the same attitude among the oral and maxillofacial surgeons and anesthesiologists.

While scrubbing one morning, I decided I wanted to try to blend these two areas of patient expertise. I believed it could be accomplished if I had an RN degree. I could then appreciate and understand both sides of the medical/dental team, perhaps bridge this chasm which seemed to separate the two.

I would certainly be unique with the dual RDH/RN degrees. I'd heard of others with the same degrees but none practicing in both fields simultaneously. They either did nursing or dental hygiene. I wanted to do both!

I began to visualize how this dual degree could be offered through the university's dental hygiene curricula. Maybe a five-year program. I also thought about a rotation for hygiene students in the hospital setting during their senior year. But I put these ideas on hold while I set about obtaining my nursing degree.

A Busy Time

I was able to pursue both an associate's degree in nursing and an RN degree at a local community college. All my previous dental hygiene credits were transferable; I needed only the clinical nursing courses and it would take two years.

Hectic times lay ahead. I soon found myself in the throes of an ill-timed divorce which sapped some of my energy but none of my enthusiasm. I still maintained my position with the university as well as participate in intramural faculty practice of dental hygiene one evening a week and Saturdays. All this while locating a new residence and studying to do well academically!

The university administrators and my colleagues were extremely supportive and gave me unlimited flexibility and encouragement. Without this support I could never have accomplished the monumental task before me.

After my nursing studies in the morning, I was back at the university or in the OR in the afternoon. Here I could apply all my newly-acquired knowledge immediately.

The two years went by quickly and I graduated valedictorian of my nursing class. I then did an internship for several months in the open heart surgery step-down unit at the university hospital. This experience gave me the opportunity to experience full-time nursing.

Making the Combination Work

I soon resumed my full-time position back at the university and began to see other hospitalized patients as well as those in oral and maxillofacial and orthognathic surgery.

Trauma and stroke patients had always been a challenge, but now I felt confident to assess patients' needs from both hygiene and nursing levels, plan needed care based on oral and physical conditions, help coordinate the implementation of the recommended care, evaluate the therapeutic effects, and change or correct the care accordingly.

For the first time I felt I could deliver continuity of patient care to the hosptilized dental and medical patient. I had the background, and my credibility and confidence were growing steadily. I talked with doctors and nurses regarding patients and became a respected team member and colleague. The nurses and doctors became receptive to some of my ideas and incorporated many hygiene recommendations into the daily nursing care and care plans of the patients.

I provided in-service education to both the medical and nursing staffs regarding the interaction of the oral cavity with other body systems and specific patient problems, all the while working closely with my colleagues in the department of oral and maxillofacial surgery. This included all areas of oral hygiene.

I was able to do bedside dental hygiene, and initiated a senior dental hygiene hospital rotation in which the student was able to provide bedside hygiene services with the aid of a portable unit containing compressed air, water and a slow speed handpiece. (One of my ideas came off hold!)

Now I could relieve the operating room circulating nurse whose responsibilities included maintenance of patient records, positioning, medications for the patient and anesthesiologist, and communication with the other operating rooms and supervisor. This helped maintain continuity of patient care and kept the OR running at a smooth pace even during change of shifts.

In the clinics at the dental school I became involved with IV sedation and CPR training. I was able to start IV's and monitor the patients' vital signs during the surgery, and administer, under supervision, narcotic analgesics.

Each day the hours went by so quickly, there never seemed to be enough time to get everything I had planned accomplished. I reported for hospital rounds at 8 AM each morning and most often found myself still actively involved in projects at 6 or 7 PM.

The experience has been the most stimulating and challenging career opportunity in my life. I feel I'm a much better hygienist because of my nursing background and a better nurse because of my hygiene background.

The Situation Changes

After five years in this position, I remarried and my husband and I moved to a small town where he started a general dental practice.

I tried to become active in both nursing and dental hygiene but found it impossible since the dual role required proximity to a large teaching hospital. Local oral and maxillofacial surgeons do few orthognathic surgery cases and can't afford the luxury of a "hybrid" RDH/RN.

I took a full-time position in the OR at the local hospital and worked there for several years in all areas of surgery both as a circulating and scrub nurse.

I am now employed as a chairside RDH in my husband's practice where I've been able to adapt and utilize many of the aseptic and sterile techniques I learned in the OR. These are especially helpful to all of us in the practice, since we are challenged by patients who may present for treatment with hepatitis, are HIV-positive or have AIDS.

Knowledge of current medication and their interactions, management of dental emergencies, manifestation of systemic disease and being a patient advocate are but a few of the nursing functions I put to use on a daily basis while practicing dental hygiene.

Is it For You?

Would you like to do it? You can! You can make nursing and hygiene tailor-made for yourself. See what requirements are needed for enrollment toward a nursing degree by your local community college. Look into part-time attendance and scholarship aid. Most of all, make the effort. It's worth it!

Working as an RDH/RN may not be the area which appeals to everyone, but I've found it a most dynamic and challenging opportunity, one in which I grow every day, one which will always hold my interest. I am glad I followed my desire.

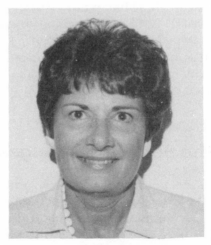

Mary Y. Holston

RDH Working Abroad

A Guide to Working Abroad

You see an ad in one of your professional journals or magazines for an RDH to work in a private dental practice in Germany, Italy, or Switzerland. You think, "Why not? I've always wanted to travel. It's the right time in my life to be looking at another kind of work environment. Why not work abroad? I might not know the language but I know dental hygiene. How difficult can it be to do the same work in another country? Yes," you decide, "I'm definitely going to look into it." Your excitement builds up and you send off your résumé.

You get the job and your correspondence with the doctor assures you there will be modest, affordable housing waiting for you and a salary that sounds pretty good. He wants you to start in two months. Now what do you do? What will you need in the way of documentation? Information? Where do you start?

Where to Begin

Passports: Every American citizen who travels abroad needs a valid U.S. passport. It's the best documentation you can have while traveling overseas and usually required to depart or enter the United States and most foreign countries.

If you're a first-time applicant, you must apply in person at a passport agency (located in major cities), authorized clerk of court (Hall of Records in your county courthouse), or a main post office to fill out an application (Form DSP-11).

Bring with you proof of U.S. citizenship (i.e., a certified copy of a birth certificate or a certificate of naturalization or citizenship), two identical, recent, front-view photographs with a light background (2" × 2"), proof of identity (i.e., a valid driver's license). Be prepared to pay $65.00 for a 10-year adult passport.

If you already have a passport (issued within the past 12 years and after your 16th birthday), you can apply by mail. Simply pick up the form (DSP-82) which is available at most courthouses and many post offices or travel agencies. Fill it out and send it to a passport agency with your old passport, two new photos, and fee of $55.00. Your new passport will be mailed to you in about six weeks.

Visas: Necessary visas should be obtained before proceeding abroad. To find out if you need a visa (since you'll be staying longer than the usual tourist/business few months), contact the country's embassy or consulate here in the United States for the most up-to-date information on visa requirements. You can also ask your travel agent, or send 50 cents with your request for the booklet, "Foreign Entry Requirements," to the Consumer Information Center, Pueblo, CO 81009. In this informative publication each country outlines what is required for entry. (Also included are names and addresses of each country's embassy, consulate or mission.)

You'll probably find out you need a working visa or permit. These are usually good for a period of one or two years. However, you will need proof of employment. Your new employer/dentist can assist you in your visa requirements. That person then becomes your sponsor.

Immunizations: Under the International Health Regulations adopted by the World Health Organization, a country may require International Certificates of Vaccination against yellow fever. A few countries still require a cholera immunization as well. Check with your medical doctor or your own records to ensure other immunizations (e.g. tetanus and polio) are up-to-date. Prophylactic medication for malaria and certain other preventive measures are advisable for some travelers. No immunizations are required to return to the United States.

Pertinent information is included in "Health Information for International Travel," available for $5 from the Superintendent of Documents, U.S. Government Printing Office, Washington, D.C. 20402 (202/783–3238). You can also check with your local health department, physician or the Centers for Disease Control at 404/639–2572 to find out about publication availability.

Bear in mind that an increasing number of countries have established regulations regarding AIDS testing, particularly for long-term visitors. (In Germany, for example, applicants for Bavaria residency permits for over 180 days require AIDS testing. The U.S. test is not accepted; in Australia, it is.) Check with the embassy or consulate of the country you'd like to work in to verify if this is a requirement for entry.

Credentials for Working: Photocopy your degrees, certificates and your license(s). Send them to your future employer. No advanced courses should be needed unless you want to take a language course for the country you will be working in.

Recommendations from present employers, hygiene school instructors, religious leader and character references from your friends should be sufficient references.

You should have at least two or three years' working experience here in the states before applying for overseas work. Some countries even have a minimum age requirement for guest workers.

Be sure to have several passport-sized black and white photographs of yourself available. They might be needed for all the necessary

119

paperwork. The same goes for your résumé. A physical examination might be required.

Going as a Vistor First

A good way to check out a country for working options is to vacation there. As a visitor, go to the American Embassy for information, query the local dental societies for prospective employers, see if there's a local dental hygiene association which could answer your questions on the cost of housing, food and the going salary level.

Check travel costs for excursions, and the local income tax (if any) that must be paid to that government. Most countries have an income tax for their guest workers. (Switzerland, England and Italy do.)

Ask the service personnel in the hotel you're staying in who they recommend for guests who need emergency dental treatment. Then call that doctor to ask for assistance in your quest for job information. Investigating all these possibilities will give you first-hand information on living conditions and job opportunities.

If You Didn't Answer an Ad

Now let's say you didn't respond to an ad (or did but it didn't work out) and are interested in working abroad. Only you're not sure in which country you want to work. Not a problem. The American Dental Hygienists' Association and the U.S. Government publish information to help you decide.

The publication, "ADHA's Foreign Employment Listing" is filled with names and addresses of contact people and organizations in Canada, Europe, the United Kingdom, Australia, New Zealand, Scandinavia, etc. (A listing from an American Dental Association publication is included; however, it did not reproduce well. For accurate addresses, get the directory directly from the ADA. See below for both organizations' phone numbers.)

Of great value in the ADHA publication are descriptions of several countries' licensing requirements, information on how to apply for work permits, what the duties of a dental hygienist in that country are, whether or not RDHs operate under direct or indirect supervision and other such pertinent information. This resource is a must for any hygienist considering working abroad. Call the ADHA at 312/440–8900 to find out the price and availability of their foreign employment listing; call the ADA at 312/440–2500 for the cost of "National and International Dental Organizations of the World."

A useful series of government publications, "Background Notes," are brief, factual pamphlets describing the countries of the world. They contain the most current information on each country's people, culture, geography, history, government, economy and political conditions. Single copies are available from the U.S. Government Printing Office. Call 202/783–3238 for pricing and ordering information.

Other Considerations

The United States will expect you to file a U.S.tax form even though you may have been out of the country a whole year. If you stay in a foreign land for 330 days out 365 and make under $75,000, you will not have to pay any U.S. income tax but you'll have to file the form anyway. Your accountant or the local IRS office will assist you with this. Or, you can get IRS publication #54, "Tax Guide for the U.S. Citizen Abroad." Many times the U.S. embassies will have American accountants there around April 15th to help the guest workers with their U.S. tax forms.

It's a good idea to register with the American Embassy once you arrive in your new country. If disaster strikes, or a war breaks out, they know their citizens are there and help them return home.

Getting to Know Yourself Better

Multi-traveler Claudine Paula Drew, who worked as an RDH in Saudi Arabia before the country became unsafe says, "The biggest single plus of living overseas is the opportunity it affords you for personal growth. You'll find you have to rely on yourself much more than usual. You won't have your usual support system, the one that buoys you up through trials and discouraging times. In becoming self-sufficent, you'll have no choice but to grow. There'll be good days; there'll be bad days. But there will never be any better days."

Bon voyage and happy growth!

RDHs in Business

Preface

Regardless of what type of business you go into, you'll have to decide what legal form of organization to use. Here are some of the rewards and drawbacks of two popular forms. (Your accountant and lawyer can be more specific. This is only the most general of information.)

Sole Proprietorship. This is the most common form a start-up business takes. As sole owner you control the business and take all the profits. These are lumped with other personal income and taxed accordingly. You can offset business losses against your personal income.

No legal formalities are required (other than what your state requires when you register your business), and it's easy to start up or close down the business. Bookkeeping, tax and legal problems generally are relatively simple.

The greatest drawback is that you are personally responsible for all debts and your personal assets can be at risk. That liability puts a limit on the amount of capital you can borrow, so expansion may depend largely on reinvested profits.

Partnership. This consists of two or more owners, perhaps including general (managing) and limited (investors) partners. One advantage of a partnership is that more people can invest in the business using personal assets as collateral for loans. They can also contribute expertise to various aspects of running the enterprise.

Partners are taxed in the same way as sole proprietors, and general partners are both individually and collectively liable for the partnership's debts and other partner's actions.

Unless you and your partners get along, the arrangement may make eveyone miserable. If one partner dies or withdraws from the business, the partnership is terminated. The other partner may then have to buy out that partner's share or find a buyer who wants to become a partner.

Ask your accountant to expound on these two forms of ownership and which—of all the variations available—is best for you.

It should be clear there's a lot of homework to be done before you start your own business. Some say the first step lies in asking yourself, "Do I have what it takes to be an entrepeneur?" Studying the characteristics of successful business owners will help you tell whether your personality traits, experiences and values are similar to those who have succeeded. Assessing your experience, skills and life goals will also help you decide if you want to invest the energy, time and resources that running a successful business demands.

Planning Sets the Tone

Before you make your first call looking for start-up capital—whether it's from family, friends or a lending agency—you must have a plan. Your plan should answer these questions:

1. How big is the market for my product or service? Who exactly will buy it and why do they need it?

2. How will I reach them and persuade them to buy it? (The best product in the world is worth nothing if people don't realize they need it.)

3. How much money do I need?

4. How long will I need it for?

5. When and how will I pay it back?

Put your plan in writing, concisely. Putting your thoughts on paper in an orderly way convinces people. It demonstrates the seriousness with which you are approaching your decision. The document you've assembled is called a business plan. Your lawyer and accountant will help you flesh it out with short- and long-range projections. The important thing to remember is that this thought-out plan is the cornerstone upon which success is solidly built.

Doing Your Homework

The U.S. Government has a wide range of products and services to help you research and formulate your goal. Specifically, SCORE (Service Corps of Retired Executives) is a non-profit organization of retired business people who offer a consulting service at no charge. You can find them on college campuses, public libraries, through notices on bulletin boards in the post office, through the Chamber of Commerce or in the Federal listing in the phone book under "Small Business Administration." These people offer generous guidance and support and can help you organize and center your thinking and objectives. You can confide in them without feeling inadequate or foolish.

Another good source for counseling, training and financial assistance is through the Small Business Adminstration (SBA) itself. Many colleges are centers for their development offices. See if a local community college near you has one. Start with the phone book.

The SBA publishes many booklets such as "Selecting the Legal Structure for Your Business," and "Planning and Goal Setting for Small Business." Write the Small Business Administration, P.O. Box 15434, Fort Worth, TX 76119 for order form 115A which lists all the publications and processing fees.

Patent Information

If you feel you've built a better mousetrap (or toothbrush or floss holder), you should protect yourself with knowledge about how the patent process works. Patent laws, what can and cannot be patented, how to judge a patent attorney or agent and a host of other information can be found in a publication from the Patent and Trademark Office. "General Information Concerning Patents" is for sale by the Superintendent of Documents, U.S. Gov't. Printing Office, Washington, D.C. 20402. Call 202/783-3238 for pricing information or order from a government bookstore near you.

RDH as Inventor

Vonda Strong *uses her ingenuity and talent to bring a much-needed product into the hands of dental professionals.*

"I'm sorry. I know this is uncomfortable. I'll be as quick as I can." *-bzzz-* "Ok, we got it. Thank you for hanging in there for me." (Whoever invents a comfortable X-ray, I mutter, will make a million bucks!)

How many times did I say that before it occurred to me that *I* could be the one to make that million bucks? Too numerous to count! I still haven't seen that million dollar ending balance on my bank statement, but I have managed to take my simple little tissue protector—a comfort cushion—to market and live solely off its profits for the last two years.

Describing how I did it in detail would make a book in and of itself. To quote from a professional source, "The work doesn't end with just the invention. In today's world you need someone to design it, patent it, make it, label it, package it, load it, ship it, store it, advertise it, market it, distribute it, display it, explain it, sell it and deliver it." Allow me to expound on some of those verbs.

The Idea Takes Shape

One cold, fall morning during the peak of flu season, the phone rang just as I was about to leave for work. "Don't come in until 11 o'clock," instructed the office manager. "Your entire morning just cancelled."

"Hmm," I thought, "What shall I do for three hours? The house is clean, the laundry's done . . . I know! I'll explore the possibility of making those little cushions."

I let my fingers do the walking and before I knew it I had a salesman on the phone. He had foam in stock that was already known to be nontoxic. Perfect! Not only that, but when I explained that I worked in a dental office and wanted to invent a dental product, he said, "That's funny—you sound just like my hygienist!" Yep. Small world.

Next I had to find an adhesive which was already approved for skin contact and could adhere to film packets. By this time, I had already fine-tuned the shape of the tissue protector.

It was now time to file an application with the Food and Drug Administration. All such products must be registered as medical devices and manufacturing standards must be followed. Patent attorneys were working on the patent search and filing procedures. Now we needed to produce the tooling so we could make the product. Oh gosh! I needed a brochure, letterhead, order forms, shipping bags, invoices, a computer . . . MONEY!! It was all so costly. I had depleted my $20,000 capital and I was becoming an insomniac.

The next six months were extremely busy. I spent every lunch hour of my five-day work week running errands and making phone calls. Evenings and weekends were also consumed with endless tasks. As everything began to fall into place, the product was ready to be marketed. Yikes! I needed a name for the cushions! The name I had originally wanted to use was already taken. My patent attorney and graphic artist were sitting by their phones tapping fingertips on their desk tops waiting for me to decide on another name. I was standing in my operatory racking my brain while waiting for my next patient to arrive when my boss strolled into my room in his calm-humble manner and said, "How about Edge-Ease®?" I wanted to kiss him. I called the attorney, he ran the trademark search and said that it was a go! The graphic artist finished the artwork for the brochure I had designed and suddenly it all seemed so official.

Luckily for me, *Dental Products Report*, a magazine mailed to every dental office in the country printed a press release for me. It appeared on the cover of the July 1985 issue. Bingo! Orders started pouring in. The rest, as they say, is history.

Making the Transition

It was terrifying and exhilirating all at the same time. Fortunately, our profession allows us the flexibility of working as many days a week as we choose. As the business became increasingly demanding of my time, I decreased my hygiene schedule from five to four days and eventually to three. When I realized I was consistently rising at 5 AM and working until 11 PM each day in order to complete my business tasks, I knew I needed to make a change in my schedule. Eventually, after all my loans for start-up costs were paid off and I was realizing more earnings from the business than from those three days of hygiene, I knew it was time to cut the apron strings and try my efforts at running the business full time.

Even though it became obvious that the business could grow faster and be more profitable if I were able to devote my full attention to it, I was reluctant to leave dental hygiene practice. I was so fond of the dentist I worked for, the staff and many of the patients. I couldn't imagine my life without them. Once you've been in practice for a number of years and have watched those little kindergartners become high school students, those high school students become college graduates, and those college graduates marry and bring their babies into the office, it's extremely difficult to leave them and the practice knowing you will no longer be part of their lives. I still miss them all very much. However, I knew I would never be content until I tried devoting my entire effort to building my own business.

The other consideration in leaving private practice was the fear of losing that dependable paycheck. Doubts would pop into my head such as, "What if sales diminish and I quit making a profit." Then logic would kick in and say, "Look, this business has grown steadily since the first month you started. Why should it stop now?" The right and left sides of my brain had many debates.

The feeling and emotional right side said, "This is fun! It's creative and you'll enjoy marketing this. Think of all the places you'll travel to for trade shows: New York, Chicago, Miami, Las Vegas, Honolulu, San Francisco . . . places you'll never have the opportunity to visit if you practice hygiene 50 weeks a year. You'll meet new people and you can still keep in touch with the people you care about."

The analytical left brain said, "Look, if you try this and it doesn't work, you can always go back to dental hygiene practice. Meanwhile, it will be an opportunity to learn different aspects of the business, such as advertising, marketing, accounting and long-range business planning." Both sides eventually reached the same conclusion.

Reflections

I can say today that I have never regretted my decision to change career directions. I've been to all those places I mentioned and many more. My day now consists of managing one employee who handles all the direct mail marketing. We share in the shipping responsibilities and I perform the administrative and public relations duties. Now in addition to attending courses with a hygiene focus (which I continue to take in order to maintain licensure), it is common for me to attend courses on sales, advertising and management.

I wouldn't trade my dental hygiene education for anything. There is a very secure feeling knowing I have that degree. However, the business classes have broadened my education. They've made me more aware of economics, politics, and have increased my global awareness. Suddenly I'm concerned with things such as how strong the dollar is compared with the yen or the Swiss franc.

Currently, I'm trying to decide which direction I should take next with my long-range business plan. It's possible I'll seek financial support from venture capitalists and become much more aggressive with multi-media advertising campaigns. Once again there are many pros and cons to consider. I look forward to whatever the future holds.

Best wishes to all of you with your dental hygiene careers. May all your other aspirations be achieved.

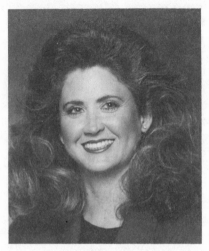

Vonda Strong

RDH in Continuing Education

Joyce Ann Turcotte *is executive director of Professional Learning Services, a company dedicated to serving the educational needs of dental professionals.*

My Background

For as long as I can remember, teaching has always been my first professional love. I enjoyed teaching my patients dental hygiene home care maintenance and the evils of periodontal disease. I found teaching dental hygiene students very stimulating, and teaching CPR to the community was also important to me.

Practicing and teaching dental hygiene for over 14 years gave me the background and confidence in my skills. Publishing articles and working in dental instrument sales added variety. Practicing in the different dental specialties further broadened my scope.

However, being an employee all my professional life was not part of my career aspirations. I function best and am most content working under my own direction. I didn't know that at first nor did I know it 15 years into my career. But I kⁿ ow it now!

Starting Up

Starting my own business, Professional Learning Services, a continuing education service for dental professionals, was the scariest yet most invigorating goal I ever set out to achieve. I didn't believe it myself.

One of my colleagues encouraged me to go on my own. She said, "If anyone can do it, it would be you." "It" meant being the only small business for dental hygiene community education in Connecticut— and who knew where else. What did I know about starting a business? Next to nothing. But when the notion took hold, I began researching the possibilities. It was a painstaking process, but in time I learned all the aspects of running my own business.

I relished the autonomy and decision making. I struggled through learning computer operations, writing a business plan, setting up an accounting system. What made building the business grow from an idea into a reality was the support structure I surrounded myself with. This fact alone made the doubtful days less doubtful and the emotionally high days fun to share. I think what made me be so unrelenting was the fear of failure. Not making it on my own.

Making the Commitment

I've been through some hard times in my life, and I discovered something about myself, especially in a crisis. I have a strong will and determination and the courage of my convictions. Some people call it "moxie;" others define it as "chutzpah" (raw nerve). I believe it is a key ingredient when the going gets tough.

I realized early on that I lacked certain business skills, so I sought expert advice from an educational consultant, accountant, business advisor, insurance agent and a lawyer to guide me through the process. Some of these experts later became members of my advisory board.

At first I wasn't sure how committed I was to the idea of starting a business. I didn't have a clue about all that was involved. A friend suggested I seek free advice from the Small Business Development Center, a federally-funded program to help assess the possibilities of becoming an entrepeneur.

I'm not shy when it comes to asking for help. There was so much to know. The small business officer discussed my ideas and asked questions to aid me in establishing a business plan and conducting a feasibility study. Through our many meetings, it was clear that this idea had potential and was worth pursuing.

It was, however, not without sweat equity. My accountant suggested bookkeeping systems and who to contact in the IRS for information. My lawyer provided me with legal guidance re contracts, copyright laws and official letters. For the first six months I spent approximately 15 hours a week researching and developing my business. Building it felt like building a sand castle—grain by grain by grain.

The research process involved studying market trends, demographics and competitors nationwide. Some of those competitors are now close networking associates with mutually beneficial business referrals and resources.

During this phase I supported myself by teaching and practicing dental hygiene. I earned no money during the research and development stage of the business and a very small profit the first year. Each subsequent year with various expansions and increased exposure via publicity, my earnings increased.

Getting Set to Go

I needed to determine the image I wanted the professional community to receive when they encountered my company. This was tough. The image came from my vision and what I thought Professional Learning Services should be and needed to be conveyed in the logo, business card and stationery. I felt that PLS should be a symbol of stability and tradition yet be on the cutting edge of what was yet to come in the profession. My husband designed the logo which I believe clearly captures the essence of my business.

At least six months before I mailed brochures, I spoke with educators and professional speakers about presenting lectures. I selected locations and met with sales staff at hotels to discuss meeting dates and costs. I worked with audiovisual specialists, caterers and hotel managers to plan every detail. Once all the details were in place, I selected a graphics design artist who could meet my price and advertising objectives.

I decided to offer a small number of continuing education seminars as a pilot project. In retrospect, this was a good move because I learned a lot from the first series of lectures without feeling overwhelmed.

I remember when I didn't take the time to do a final proofing on a brochure because I *thought* it was all set. When the 3,500 brochures were delivered and I read the top copy, I almost choked. The information that was supposed to describe one of the speakers was listed under another speaker's name! As I stapled in a correction sheet on each of the 3,500 brochures, I repeated, "You will always proof the final copy." To err is human, but when it costs time and money, it's a tragedy to the small business owner. To say the least, I learned many lessons the hard way.

Then and Now

This new business was met with resistance at first. Some competitors did what they could to undermine the work I did. Some subcontractors took advantage of my inexperience. Being the new kid on the block I took some lumps. Hindsight is 20/20 and critical for personal and professional growth. To look back at what I did, see what went wrong, know how to correct it, see what went right and know how to build on it is ultimate growth.

When I started my business endeavors I was in my first trimester of pregnancy with my son; my daughter was three years old. We were also renovating a rental property and improving our own home. I taught and practiced dental hygiene between three and four days a week. By the time I was about to deliver, I was counting the days to my first scheduled presentation. Registrations and phone calls were coming in and I remember praying to have the baby over the weekend so I wouldn't lose too much time away from the office. Believe it when I tell you that I went into labor on Friday afternoon and was back home answering calls Monday afternoon!

The business has now expanded to offer education/vacation packages, private individual and small group courses, single and multi-day conferences, and local and out-of-state refresher training programs. I am also exploring new avenues such as corporate training programs and consulting.

What Being in Business Means to Me

The greatest joys I get from owning my own business are the limitless job description, creativity, opportunity, challenge, constant learning, networking and sharing ideas. What I enjoy most is the unlimited possibilities and overall potential growth.

Having my own business allows me to set the schedule I choose most of the time, and be home with my family. Sometimes I am bruxing and clenching when I feel I'm being pulled in two, three and four directions at the same time. Having the kind of husband who is fully supportive of this undertaking is absolutely essential. Where do you get one? Only kidding!

Is Being in Business For You?

If you are thinking of starting a business, assess your capabilities and experiences in the following areas:
- Commitment
- Determination
- Perserverance
- Drive
- Opportunity and goal orientation
- Initiative
- Personal responsibility
- Problem solving ability
- Self image
- Sense of humor

- Seeking and using feedback
- Internal locus of control
- Tolerance
- Calculated risk taking
- Integrity and reliability
- Decisiveness
- Dealing with failure

This list of ''The Entrepeurial Mind'' was presented at a lecture on starting a small business sponsored by the Small Business and Development Center in my area. I consider this my working list and have referred to it many times.

Good luck!

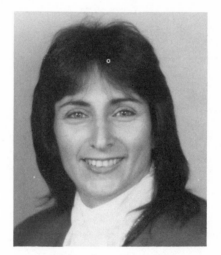

Joyce Ann Turcotte

[Readers can contact Joyce Ann Turcotte at Professional Learning Services, 31 Lois Circle, Monroe, CT 06468. Tel. 203/261-2857]

RDH in Sales

Preface

When hygienists get the urge to move out of their operatory confines, they often consider dental product sales. Here're some pointers to familiarize you with selling opportunities in the dental industry.

Retail Sales Representative: This is a form of selling directly to the end user, the dental professional. Companies marketing products either used by or dispensed through dental offices and laboratories often use this route as do local supply houses (dealers). Generally, little or no overnight travel is required as the territory to cover is fairly local. A "rep" who is employed by a dealer, often works along with manufacturer's representatives (a process called "detailing" or "co-traveling"), especially when introducing new products to practitioners.

Manufacturer's Sales Representative: A combination educator, troubleshooter and resource person who sells to dental supply houses, schools with dental programs, and government providers of dental care. Employed by companies with a field force. Entails heavy travel. It is not uncommon for a territory to extend over several states. Good salary and benefits, opportunity for bonuses, generally a company car.

Independent Sales Representative: Non-employee who represents one or more companies on a contractual basis. Can sell directly to dentists or supply houses within a proscribed territory. Popular format for multi-level marketing. Commission on sales.

What are the Pluses of Dental Products Sales?

Good situation for the do-it-myselfers, the self-starters, the ones who like to compete; the keep-moving types who enjoy being in control of their time and income; super organizers who work well with others yet like independent action. Income potential can be limitless and company benefits can be excellent.

What are the Minuses?

Long hours, many weekends spent working at conventions, lots of paperwork, rejection, and the need to be constantly organized and motivated. Stress and time management are key issues.

Requirements and Salaries

Requirements vary from company to company. With the majority of manufacturers, a degree and sales experience are necessary, but that can be waived if your bearing and demeanor appeal to the decision makers. Bear in mind that selling Mary Kay, Amway or counter sales at Christmas time well qualify as sales experience. Make a strong case for selling oral health care to patients as relevant sales background.

Depending on ability, experience and education, starting salaries for full-time work can range from the low to high twenties. In addition to salaries, commissions or bonuses can be paid on the amount of sales generated in each territory. Selling is the way to make real money through hard work if that is your goal.

Benefits are usually quite good (medical, dental, life insurance, paid vacation, etc.) and can include a company car or car allowance and travel expenses.

Is it For You?

Morris Roberts, vice president of sales for the Gel-Kam Corporation, a division of Colgate Palmolive, says, "there are great opportunities for a hygienist to succeed in sales for dental products companies. That person brings the experience and expertise of the dental professional which greatly aids these companies in marketing to the dental community."

He adds, "Even though the popular perception of a salesperson is one who is outgoing, assertive, and demonstrates a lot of energy and enthusiasm, I've had in my employ many quiet-type RDHs who were enormously successful."

Roberts has found there are three requisites necessary for successful selling: a sincere desire to satisfy other people's needs; a willingness to "expend a lot of shoe leather;" and a tenacious persistence. Along with these attributes, he adds, one has to be able to accept rejection. "For every successful sale you make," he says, "there may be as high as 20 rejections. You have to be able to deal with that."

Taking Action

Query your office's supply house representative for more information about selling as a retail representative. Ask that person to introduce you to a manufacturer's rep. Find out where the "help wanted" ads are placed, what trade publications you should be reading, who you should be sending your résumé and cover letter to.

For those whose offices are not visited by a dealer, attend the next dental convention in your area. Try to connect with one of the reps working for a company whose products interest you. (Wear a suit, whether male or female, and bring several copies of your résumé.)

For those of you working in institutions, ask the purchasing agent to advise you of the dental sales representative's next visit.

If you are a member of your state hygiene association, ask your continuing ed chairperson to invite a dental sales representative to speak at a component meeting.

Seek out sales courses offered by your local community college. Try to get selling experience even if it isn't dentally related. Read books on successful selling techniques so you're familiar with the language of sales. Take a course in public speaking to build your confidence.

Point out your efforts when you get an interview. It will clearly demonstrate your seriousness and "go-getter" attitude.

RDH in Dental Product Sales

Rebecca Van Horn *moved from clinical dental hygiene into sales and education for a major oral hygiene products manufacturer.*

Every morning when I'm home I drink coffee out of my favorite mug. The Boyton cartoon on the mug depicts a huge, hairy monster growling over a tiny, intimidated salesman who is trying to ward off this beast with his briefcase. The caption reads, "Salesmanship begins when the customer says NO!" I think about this truism every time I begin a sales presentation to a dental professional. My job is to get the customer to say YES. This, of course, is easier said than done, but there's tremendous satisfaction when the hairy beast is transformed into a kitten.

Recognizing Opportunity

I graduated from a Big Ten university in 1979. My undergraduate minor was in political science, a social science I had great interest in. I also enrolled in several women's studies course. These made me aware of current issues regarding equal opportunity in the marketplace. Since I was studying dental hygiene, a predominantly female profession, I made a promise to myself. I vowed that I would be as successful as I could be in clinical dental hygiene, but if opportunities presented themselves, I would never turn them down.

If I have three words of advice to graduating or career-changing RDHs they are these: be an opportunist. Take advantage of transfers, divorce, CTS, unemployment—whatever. Make these situations work to *your* benefit. Evaluate, contemplate, prepare and move on.

The job market in my medium-sized midwestern town was not advantageous in the early eighties. I was working two or three part-time jobs at once. Reflecting on these years, this was the time when the sales training truly began.

I worked in a local department store and I sold *everything* including lawn mowers and aluminum siding. It was really fun and made for a nice change from clinical hygiene. Then in 1985 an opportunity presented itself. My roommate lost a job and planned a move to Chicago. Did I want to go?

I had traveled to New York, Philadelphia, Boston and Chicago as I was growing up. I'm definitely a big-city person. I enjoy art museums, theatre and living in older neighborhoods with interesting architecture. So I jumped at the chance to move to Chicago, a "big town" with a reputation for being filled with friendly midwesterners.

I moved without a job. After obtaining my Illinois license, I worked as a clinical hygienist in a hospital. This was a challenging position—six different dentists to adjust to plus a large outpatient center with RNs, LPNs, therapists and physicians. The public education aspect of my job was most interesting. It prepared me for the public speaking I now use during my presentations. (Try to gain some experience in public speaking if you're interested in sales. The ability to speak and write persuasively is critical to success.)

Getting the Job

Through contacts I developed in the local hygiene association, I heard about a public relations educator position with a dental products manufacturer. I made the necessary phone calls to set up an interview. (You must be decisive and act quickly. These kinds of positions are desirable and don't stay open too long.) Within three weeks of the initial interview I was hired. A tip I learned and pass along is to always send a follow-up thank you note after an interview. It makes a good impression.

What Employers Like to See

Dental hygiene students often ask me how I found my niche in the dental industry, what qualities employers are looking for, and whether a business education is necessary for sales.

I always tell them that although a bachelor's degree in business may help one understand the direction of a company, it is not essential for a sales position. However, if someone wants to pursue a marketing job within a company, then I would encourage that person to study business.

A knowledge of the products a company sells, previous retail selling experience (or telemarketing), a bachelor's degree and the ability to speak and write confidently and professionally are probably some requisites to consider. At a certain administrative level within the organization, an MBA might help move you ahead.

I had been a clinical hygienist for seven years in both private practice and a hospital setting before I was hired for my present position. Employers like to see a variety of clinical practice settings on your résumé. It tells them you're flexible, that you adapt well to new situations. This is critical in sales because you are constantly adapting—no two days are ever the same. You're constantly traveling around to different clients. There's no 9 to 5 routine; *you* set your own schedule. Many companies allow you to work out of your home with computer and fax link-ups and car phones.

My current employer was also interested in my previous sales experience. Had I ever sold anything? Of course. As hygienists, don't we sell oral health to our patients every day? In addition to this, consider pursuing some part-time sales (in anything) while you're doing clinical hygiene. My reasoning for this is you'll be better at understanding what benefit-feature selling technique is in addition to developing a "thick skin." (Benefit-feature selling is convincing the customer of the benefit of the product or service you're selling *before* you discuss the actual features or characteristics of the product. If customers see the benefits first, they'll buy from you.)

It's important to develop a "thick skin" as you do part-time sales. You'll hear many NOs out there, but you can't let that get under your skin. You must be enthusiastic, helpful and assertive. And never take NO as the final answer. It means being persistent, calling and following up.

The buzz word in today's business-sales world is customer service. We are less in the business of persuasion than in servicing accounts in whatever ways it takes to keep them satisfied.

Product knowledge is essential. Think about the last time you didn't buy something because the salesperson couldn't answer basic questions about the item. Most companies today provide initial training about the products when you're hired. Then there will be follow-up seminars as new products are introduced.

It's also important to know your competitors' products if you want to sell effectively against them. *Dental Products Report*, a publication mailed free to dental offices nationwide, is read widely in the industry because it provides solid information on the newest dental products. You have to understand your marketplace and the people (dental office personnel) who work in this arena every day. Their needs create the demand for your products.

What I Do

My particular position today is part sales, part educator. I sell quality dental products to decision makers in dental and dental hygiene schools. All companies in this industry want their products used by students. Hopefully, future professionals will use the same products in their offices after graduation. Name recognition is important. It is easier to sell products familiar to professionals than it is to sell those from upstart companies.

The other responsibility I have is presenting quality slide presentations to students and continuing education groups. In these presentations you can't be too commercial, especially in the schools. You're there to educate, not so much to sell.

Many companies believe these types of programs are important because they provide support for their product lines. I truly enjoy the lecturing. It helps keep me current with the literature.

Salaries and Benefits

Sales positions today, in general, pay about the same initially as a full-time dental hygiene clinical position in a private practice (except in high-paying areas like California). The difference can be at bonus time. Here there is an opportunity to earn considerably more money if you are more energetic and ambitious. It really is up to you if you'd like to earn more. This aspect of sales always appealed to me. I like to have more control over what my annual income is than is possible with clinical practice.

Salespeople appear to have glamorous jobs. As a clinical hygienist, I was always impressed with our manufacturer representatives for this reason. I have since learned that an essential part of convincing your customer is looking the part. Your personal appearance must evoke confidence and be professional. You should always look good even though inside you might not feel this way. This is a job challenge all salespeople encounter.

Overnight and weekend travel is inevitable with many lonely nights away from home. This is balanced by the chance to visit new places you might never have traveled to on your own.

Most larger companies today consider a company car a taxable benefit along with full health coverage, life and travel insurance, a pension plan and tuition reimbursement.

A sales position within the dental care industry offers a hygienist the opportunity to expand upon his or her clinical knowledge and to challenge him or herself on a daily basis. As the marketplace becomes more competitive, with increased pressure from foreign manufacturers and larger companies, the knowledge and energy many RDHs have (but feel they are not utilizing) will be necessary in a sales position.

Develop contacts with the representatives who visit your office. They usually know when vacancies exist. Let all your colleagues know you're interested in a sales position. The word will get around. Companies are always looking for the best-qualified applicant. Spend your time now becoming the best qualified for your next career opportunity.

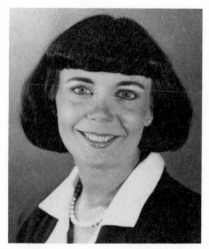

Rebecca Van Horn

Second Time Around: Re-Entry into Dental Hygiene

An RDH Re-Enters Hygiene

Ann Flynn Scarff *presents her view of what makes dental hygiene special enough for her to return to it.*

Where I Came From

I feel like the television comic who says, "Baseball has been velly, velly good to me." Dental hygiene has been very, very good to me. It has allowed me to practice in four states, teach a variety of related subjects, edit two state association newsletters, develop new skills in dental hygiene assessment, care planning and presentation, treatment and evaluation, and has given me the security to leave it while trying another career. Now I've returned to private practice.

I left hygiene in 1983 when a friend's computer company needed a non-technical trainer and salesperson. What an opportunity that turned into! I am one of those easily trainable people who enjoys a challenge, and I always thought I'd be good in the business world. I wanted to try my hand at being both an entrepeneur and a salesperson. This was a startup company looking for a non-engineer who could learn their computer graphics system and provide input for their users' manuals.

I soon found that my people skills worked well at trade shows where I could handle crowds and demonstrate and present some complicated technical information. Over the next seven years I merged dedication to the job, long hours and frustration with the excitement of bringing a great product to market. These qualities, all second nature to an RDH, are great credentials for trying a new line of work. After all, I reasoned, what did I have to lose? I always had my hygiene license to fall back on.

In small companies everybody does everything, so my experience was varied. I eventually left that company for another where I was sales director for one component of the graphics system. I'm a good self-motivator, so activities requiring organization and management soon followed.

However, sales tend to be competitive and isolating. These qualities bothered me. I really enjoy collegiality. I was astonished to see that many salespeople do not share their discoveries and techniques.

Meanwhile, I landed some major contracts for computer products, called on most high tech and large businesses in northern California, and opened a regional office for a Texas manufacturer. I traveled all over the country, handled personalities from engineers to company presidents, and learned to sell some very technical computer devices.

These activities can be stressful, so I was not surprised when my hygienist friend found 5mm pockets all over my mouth. She sent me to a periodontist. I was mortified to discover I was clenching and neglecting my own mouth in this fury of the business world.

After seven years, I was getting tired of the razzle-dazzle, constant travel and high pressure of sales. A recession was starting in northern California and I was losing my enthusiasm for selling expensive products to a business community that wanted to tighten their budgets. When a big project went sour after three months of effort, I decided to retire from that business and take a few months to figure out what I would do next. It never occurred to me at the beginning of my reflections that I'd be back in dental hygiene. But I am one of those people who believes my instincts and environment direct me. They led me back to the original training and interests I had as a young student over 25 years ago.

How I Returned

I credit my network of dental hygiene friends with pointing the way. After two months of enjoying my free time, I became obsessed with two things: a software program that led to newsletter production, and baking bread. That may seem a long way from Gracey curets, but they are related.

Baking is a wonderful, physical activity. The excitement of new flavors, new feel of ingredients, new smells from the oven and new taste is appreciated by everyone—especially me! I enjoy great breads and bakers, but running a bakery is too time-consuming, unprofitable and the hours are too long.

Newsletters, however, are both fun and easy. I designed one as a Christmas present for my sisters in which I gave away all my baking secrets. But publishing like this is usually volunteer work and would not pay the rent. I kept asking myself what I could do that would allow me to work with my hands, provide lots of intellectual stimulation, be profitable, and keep me out of the overwork syndromes I migrate toward.

It was serendipitous that a hygiene friend asked me to substitute for her in a dental practice where I had once worked. At first I said no because so much had changed in the seven years I'd been away: infection control . . . therapeutic root planing . . . more perio recall in general practice. But I did know and enjoy the practice. It was familiar to me. It would be a perfect re-entry.

The butterflies started as soon as I said yes. I ignored my concerns with the (unfounded) belief that as a former teacher, I was better qualified than the average substitute hygienist. My misconception about this got me going, although in reality, I now know I was not up to par those first few days.

My Initial Reactions

What I enjoyed first was the patient contact. I get something unique from each patient. Often a new dental condition provides an insight into the personality before me. Sometimes it's a view into the human condition; othertimes it's social commentaries on health issues, politics or patient concerns.

I found that staying on time was easier when my skills were a little rusty than when I remembered all the things I used to do during an appointment. Staying on time is still a challenge for me and it may always be so because of the nature of providing services. But my experience in sales was an insight into how essential time management is to running a good business. I have new respect for the dental practitioner who is operating a good, professional business.

However the biggest surprise about returning to practice was the good feeling at the end of the day that I had provided eight to 10 patients with a complete assessment of their oral hygiene, provided appropriate treatment or referral, and could now collect a check and return home with no problems or carry-over to the next day. No more arguing with sales managers over every little point of commission due. This felt like recreation compared to the last seven years!

I had to get serious with myself and admit that 1) dental hygiene is a valuable contribution to society; 2) I have a good foundation and am good at my profession; 3) I am real comfortable in the dental office and value the teamwork of a good dental practice; 4) a lot of business is just "busy work" that leads to other work and more jobs, but my instincts and philosophy of life have returned to preserving the environment, not making more work out of something simple; and 5) these values had opened up more activities that I wanted to do with my free time than work long hours. At age 46, it takes time to take care of myself and I know that's well-invested time.

Regaining My Professional Skills

Getting back into the profession was not that easy, however. My next call was to a local employment agency where they asked for the appropriate licensing information. When I had changed my California license to retired status in 1985, I understood that I would not have to take continuing education credits until the year I chose to return to active status. The agencies told me the rules had changed. I now had to take those 25 credits *before* they would activate my license! I apologized to my friend for practicing illegally and set about getting CEUs.

I was fortunate. In six weeks I had them all. I found a two-day course on local anesthesia which allowed me to practice my old skills in an educational setting. I got recertified in CPR (the long course), so my confidence was reestablished in life support and emergencies.

Infection control was an area where I definitely needed new education. When last seen in the office, I was swabbing everything with alcohol. Now I understand the advantages of many different products and can recommend a variety of disinfectants and sterilization procedures to patients and office personnel. I use ultrasound to remove debris from instruments so as not to stick myself. I maintain instrument sharpness by drying them well before putting them in the chemical autoclave, or use an anti-oxidant bath before steam autoclave. (I am constantly astonished at the number of offices which have faulty sterilization procedures.)

Other areas I have added to my new dental hygiene education are procedures for care of implants. I can recognize and maintain the new restorative materials that were not around seven years ago. Oral pathology has gotten much more complex since the eighties, but I find continued learning in our profession to be as fascinating as it was in 1966.

Preventing Burnout

Burnout is not a new phenomenon to me. For instance, my sales career was not short-lived, but once I had achieved the healthy $65,000 salary plus benefits, I was ready to change because the repeated challenge of having another good month was not a unique experience. I had had enough of that. And even my teaching experience had me under publishing pressure that felt uncomfortable with my other goals. I feel well-rounded when I exercise daily, take vacations, spend lots of time with my family and friends, learn a little, and experience new things regularly. Jobs that prohibit these things don't work for me. They once did but my life and philosophies have changed.

I made another wise decision and called on my former boss, the director of the dental hygiene program where I had worked. She brainstormed with me about what else besides teaching was out there for me. We discussed her upcoming textbook and the meeting ended up with me agreeing to contribute a chapter to it. Interestingly, compensation for this task was not my goal; catching up with what had happened in hygiene the past few years was.

I conquer burnout with new challenges. Researching and writing my chapter took me to the medical school library for months. I wrote and learned and re-learned the foundation of our practice. I now subscribe to several publications I consider essential for staying abreast and interested in dental hygiene.

For me, attending component meetings is much more than networking and continuing education courses. It is having a say in and control over my practice through legislation, communication and the democratic process. I am really proud of how the California Dental Hygienists' Association has kept our profession protected from attempts at preceptorship and licensure of dental students as dental hygienists. We have expanded functions of local anesthesia, nitrous oxide/oxygen anesthesia and soft tissue curettage in my state. This was hard fought for legislation that provides me with more challenge to my practice. I want to know the reasons our laws change, what the controversial issues are, and what other RDHs think and feel. I get these from the CDHA.

My Working Conditions

It's wonderful to be a middle-aged RDH with all these experiences who can easily support herself and still have a whole life outside the office. Compatible professional values with my employers is an important job requirement for me. I am currently working 1½ days per week for one excellent general dentist and one day for another. Both are real special in that their care for patients is carefully thought-out. I have referred friends to both of them with full confidence.

I am regularly developing better systems with the other RDHs in one practice, and in the other, I am helping to establish a new dentist who really appreciates good dental hygiene. (She practiced as an RDH for several years before starting her dental practice.)

The area I live in has four dental hygiene placement agencies. In the manpower shortage of today, I can work nearly any day I choose with a guaranteed salary of $225 to $230 per day. I am always surpised that a dentist will offer me a job without even evaluating my philosophies and even sometimes without evaluating my work! They are that desperate for a dental hygienist. It's interesting to be part of our profession at a time when we are in such great demand and expect proper working conditions.

I must admit I feel evangelical about insisting on good working conditions. Maybe it's my chance to convert dentistry to respecting good infection control, proper instruments, adequate appointment time, and smooth appointment flow in the practice. Since I pick up an extra day or two each week, I use every opportunity to tell employers about how it is done well in other offices. This variety gives me the challenges I need in my work environment.

Looking Back

It was really simple and direct to make this career change. Re-entering dental hygiene came at the right time and the right place for me. There were times when my hands and back ached and I wondered if I could do it again. Then I remembered that no one was born with a curet in his or her hand, and that I could get in shape to do this just as I did 26 years ago.

I have not regretted my choice, and I do not foresee, right now, my satisfaction with private practice changing any time soon. I do expect it to mature and become better and better. I plan to share some of the assessment styles I learned in researching the book chapter with my local component. After all, hygienists are my people and I learn at least as much from sharing my experiences as I do from hearing theirs. I do enjoy being a hygienist again!

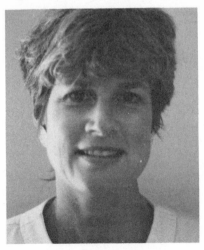

Ann Flynn Scarff

Résumés That Get
the Interview

How to Write an Effective Résumé

Q. What's the purpose of a résumé?

A. To get an interview.

Yes, the primary purpose of a résumé is to get you that all-important interview, that special encounter where you and a prospective employer size each other up, see if what you offer is in keeping with what he or she is looking for; the place where you both decide if it's a "go."

Many RDHs think they don't need a résumé. "After all," they reason, "an employer knows what I am licensed to do. Why do I have to put it in writing? Why can't I just tell him or her face-to-face about my experience?" And for those new graduates who may be on the short end of experience, what good will a résumé do them?

In a word, plenty. A résumé is more than a listing of jobs with dates and places worked. It is a written demonstration of your organizational skills, your market savvy, the accomplishments you've achieved to date. It positions you clearly in prospective employers' minds so that they know what makes you special *before* you appear. Interviews are not the time for surprises. That's what you sometimes get when you're only working from a voice on the telephone. Forwarding a résumé in advance of the interview makes sure the image being visualized is the one you want that person to have.

In today's tight job market, hygienists are in the unique position of being in demand and commanding respectable salaries. To be on the cutting edge of this enviable footing, you have to market yourself professionally. This means a well-crafted résumé, an approach used routinely in both business and the professions.

Identify Your Objective

Start with identifying your job objective. If you want to work in a specialty practice, say so up front, as in, "Dental Hygienist in a High-Quality Periodontics Practice," or, "Dental Health Educator in a Community-based Medical/Dental Clinic." This way everybody—including you—knows what your goal is. If nothing else, it helps you stay focused as you think through your qualifications.

Here are some job objectives submitted by RDHs. Which do you think would influence a prospective employer to interview the person?

A. To apply the knowledge of my education and experience toward the growth and improvement of oral health.

B. Periodontal therapist in a general dental practice. I am an enthusiastic communicator, sincere and friendly in relating to people.

C. To obtain a position that will enable me to use my creative, analytic and written skills to foster personal and professional growth.

D. I am presently attending a health services management program. I am seeking a position as a dental administrator.

Do you see how much stronger and purposeful items B and D are? Office managers, department heads, administrators and other people in decision-making positons are not career counselors. They don't have the time or skill to figure out where your talents could best be used in their organization. Their job is to decide *if* you fit, not where.

New Graduate

A new graduate could consider these two job objectives:

1. After receiving licensure, my desire is to work as a dental hygienist in a prevention-oriented general practice.

2. My professional objective is to use my expanded functions training within the clinical setting in either a private dental office or a public health facility.

It is important to identify your job objective right up front. It establishes the way you see yourself professionally in the receiver's mind.

Chronological or Functional?

The chronological format flows backward, job by job, year by year, with the most recent position listed first. It is a familiar style to employers as it outlines your work history.

The functional résumé relays accomplishments in skill areas by highlighting what you have done (as opposed to where and when you have done it). If your employment history is limited, if it includes a lot of volunteer work, if you've been out of the job market a while, or if you're thinking of shifting to another arena of oral health care, the functional style may work as a better tool for you.

Whichever style you use, show a continuing progression of marketable skills and experience which leads to your present job objective. Do this under the next category, experience.

What is Your Experience?

Shape your experiences, both paid and voluntary, to fit your job objective. For example, if you are going for a position that involves administrative tasks—like an office manager or clinic coordinator—zero in on your organizational skills. Give your clinical responsibilities a lower profile.

Wrong: "Purchased clinical supplies."

Right: "Changed ordering and inventory control system to achieve a 20 percent cost reduction."

Wrong: "Volunteer, handicapped children."

Right: "I planned and supervised an oral health program for 30 handicapped children, their parents and two nurses over a six-month period. Follow up showed an 80 percent increase in improved home care."

Wrong: "Made crafts for our church/component/school health fair."

Right: "I made crafts which netted the organization $700 in a two-day sale."

In the clinical context, did you "Plan treatments and provide complete prophylaxes" (responsibility only), or did you "Initiate a patient education program which reduced the rate of gingival inflammation by two-thirds (identifies achievement and problem-solving skills)?"

Did you "change the recall system" or did you "revamp the recall system so that patient visits were increased by 27 percent from the previous year?"

Whenever possible, emphasize the successful results you achieved. Talk about the amount of money raised or saved, the number of people who used the service or product, the satisfaction expressed by those for whom the activity was undertaken or the action that evolved as a result of your efforts.

Now your prospective employer knows what you can do (did!), what value you will be to him or her. The information you're giving is results oriented. It shows you know how to solve problems.

The Right Words

Use action words, ones that connote authority, such as initiated, handled, supervised, coordinated, designed, planned. These verbs always take an object and imply a result (initiated *what*? handled *what*? supervised *whom*?)

Stay away from the passive voice, as in "responsibilities included . . ." For example, "Fourteen new dental hygienists were recruited by me for our local component" is considerably less effective than "I initiated a recruitment program for our local hygiene component which resulted in 14 new members, bringing our membership to one of the highest in the state. I am now chairperson of the state membership committee."

If you worked with others on a particular project, use terms such as co-authored, co-led, rather than the weaker sounding "helped write," "helped lead."

Good work that produces results doesn't need embellishment through overstuffed language to get its message across. And don't be afraid to use the pronoun, "I." Who else did these things?

A note of caution: While suggesting you describe your experience as impressively as possible, no way should you lie about what you have done. The distinction is important and should not be forgotten. Your goal is to develop an honest and effective "sales pitch" about your experiences to sell yourself for jobs you are authentically qualified to perform.

Even if you are a new graduate, you probably have had some experience during your training that led you to enjoy one aspect of hygiene over another. If that was not the case, draw from your work experiences in life, both paid and voluntary, and shape them to fit your job objective. If nothing in your background seems relevant, highlight your education instead of bringing your lack of experience into the limelight.

Education, Honors and Awards

Now is the time to list all your academic achievements (especially top of the class), honors and awards. If you've received specific recognition, presented table clinics, or participated in or led accredited continuing education courses, identify them.

Some new graduates list their extramural training and professional activities within the school context right after their entry on education. It's a good idea as it positions the writer in the receiver's eyes as an involved person, even if experience is on the short side.

Personal Data

Here is the place to say, "excellent health," "available for travel" (if it relates to your job objective and is true), "references on

159

request," "salary negotiable" and mention your hobbies and other interests.

You are not required to indicate your marital status, number of children or age. Some people use this section to make a values statement such as, "I am a concerned health care professional, dedicated, involved and eager to accept new challenges." Come across as a well-rounded individual with a personality as well as abilities.

Format

People tend to think there is a single way in which to form the information on their résumés. Not so. Your job objective and statements backing it up are your priority items and should be paramount. If that means highlighting your work experience ahead of your education, so be it. If you are a new graduate with limited experience, lead with your academic accomplishments. It's the *focus* that's important. Whatever your structure, try to keep the sentences short and tight.

Your name, address and phone number should hit the eye first. Use quality white or off-white paper on a computer or use offset printing. No cheap duplicating paper or dot-matrix printing.

Single spacing with wide margins on both sides and bottom is easy to read. Check for grammatical errors and misspellings. Get someone else to review it. Keep the length to 1½ pages.

Who Gets the Job?

Jobs do not go to people with the longest résumés written in the most eloquent language based on inflated experiences. The best test is that you can talk about anything on your résumé with ease. Remember, its purpose is to get you an interview.

And don't forget the person reading your résumé. Make it easy for him or her to say, "This applicant knows what she wants and what she can deliver."

See the following examples for suggested résumé styles.

New Graduate

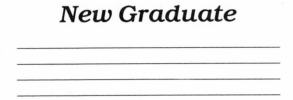

JOB OBJECTIVE
Dental Hygienist in a pediatric dentistry practice

EDUCATION
Bachelor of Science, May 1991, Southern Illinois University, Carbondale, Illinois

Major: Dental Health Care Management and Promotion

Associate in Art, May 1990, SIU

Major: Dental Hygiene

Attended Quincey College, 1986–1988, Quincey, IL

EXPERIENCE
1986–1988 Student Office Manager at Quincey College Admissions Office

Externship, SIU Mobile Dental Facility. Serviced rural areas in southern Illinois.

Externship, SIU Dental School, Alton, IL. Included working at the East St. Louis Dental Clinic and St. Mary's Hospital.

Externship, Veterans Hospital, Marion, IL.

HONORS AND ACTIVITIES
Dean's List, five semesters; member of Sigma Phi Alpha (National Dental Hygiene Honor Society); SADHA; President of Interhall (major campus organization); Student Welfare Organization representative; IL Congress of Parents and Teachers Association Vocational Scholarship; American Legion Scholarship; Henry Bunn Memorial Scholarship.

Presented a table clinic on "Stress and TMJ" at an SIU health fair. Planned and implemented a dental health program for a sixth grade class at Lewis School, Carbondale, IL.

PERSONAL DATA
Excellent health, single, references on request.

New Graduate

JOB OBJECTIVE

Dental Hygienist in a general practice. I am especially skilled with geriatric patients.

EDUCATION

Certificate in Dental Hygiene

Associate in Applied Science
The University of Medicine and Dentistry,
Newark, NJ   December 1990

LICENSURE

Northeast Regional Board Certificate   1991
New Jersey Dental Hygiene License   current
CPR certification   current

EXPERIENCE

Dental Assistant, private practice   1988–1989

Assisted in general dentistry, periodontology, oral surgery. This job enabled me to become familiar with and experienced in different dental specialties.

Machine Operator, XYZ company   1986–1988

Took leadership in a work group of eight people. This role enabled me to organize strategies for high production and gave me the ability to lead people toward a common goal.

PERSONAL DATA

Practice philosophy:

I believe in delivering quality care to my patients. I believe in strong infection control policies, disease prevention and my role in both. I believe in continuing my education and expanding my knowledge to be the best dental hygienist I can be.

Personal philosophy:

I am an excellent team member who gets along well with people. I am quick at catching on to procedures, am a hard worker and eager to accept a challenge. References available upon request.

Experienced: Clinical

CAREER GOAL

To work in an environment which enhances my personal as well as team growth; to give quality dental care to clients through the use of my clinical and communication skills. I believe in co-diagnosis between the health care provider and the individual. This allows people to realize their own needs which in turn encourages them to maintain good oral health.

In the past five years I have been involved in a hygiene-driven, teams-monitored dental wellness practice. The following is a list of some of the functions I assisted with:

EXPERIENCE

• Initiation of a soft tissue management program for individuals with disease characteristics ranging from gingivitis to rapidly progressive periodontal problems to where I received a 90% acceptance rate.

• Increased hygiene production to almost 300%.

• Maintained and supported 90% of moderate to advanced periodontal cases with non-surgical techniques, with the result that clients avoided surgery and had a 2–5mm pocket reduction.

• Evaluated and treatment planned 95% of periodontal cases. This reduced stress for the dentist.

• Developed, coordinated and implemented a working recall system to the point where a second hygienist was needed.

• Responsibility for daily input of clients on the computer regarding their fees, appointments, pre-treatment plans, treatment notes and insurance forms.

• Began each day by being on time, organizing charts and coordinating therapy between hygiene and treatment coordinators.

• Utilization of a phase microscope as a diagnostic, educational and motivational tool in

163

order to get the client more involved in his or her own therapy.

• Marketed the practice by building relationships with my clients and being empathetic to their personal and oral health needs.

• Supplied oral hygiene tools to the individual according to that person's dexterity and motivational needs.

• Currently, I am maintaining (therefore bonded) financial records for a professional organization with an annual membership of 400 and an operating budget of $20,000. I attend meetings, compose letters, coordinate phone calls and handle issues on a local and national level.

EDUCATION AND CREDENTIALS

B.S., West Liberty State College, West Virginia

Registered Dental Hygienist, Pennsylvania and Arizona

Certified in Local Anesthesia

Certified in Basic Life Support

Licensed in Expanded Functions in Periodontics

Member, ADHA and Arizona DHA

Member of the Western Society of Periodontology

Member of the Western Regional Examining Board

Over 60 CEUs acquired annually

REFERENCES

Complete list upon request.

Experienced: Manager

OBJECTIVE   FINANCIAL COORDINATOR with a health care organization. I am a positive, strong communicator with a good feel for handling people.

Professional Experience

August 1984–Present   Dental financial coordinator for a large family dental center.

Administration: Reduced accounts receivable by eliminating billing department. This was accomplished through the consolidation of computerizing individualized recordkeeping of insurance paid and patient's obligation.

Instituted a career ladder training program for 50 business assistants. As workers' skills and confidence increased, they were promoted to the next step.

Designed and implemented a financial curriculum via self-programmed instruction for professionals and assistants within the facility. This curriculum provided for continuing education.

Supervision: Supervised and trained 12 business assistants in all financial procedures of facility.

Coordinated and managed all billing procedures as they related to patient flow and reimbursement.

October 1979–July 1984   Dental hygienist and business assistant in private practice.

Established a recall system to improve and increase patient contact. There was a 35% increase in patient return for preventive care.

Initiated a patient education program with the result that there was a significant reduction in the gingival inflammation index and a lowering of the DMF rate in the child patient population.

Prior to 1979   Professional work was part time as dental hygienist in private practice as family responsibilities were primary.

Related Experience

Bingo coordinator for religious institution
  —Group leader for 25 people involved in executing program
  —Bookkeeper
  —Handle all money transactions
  —Monitor legal aspects
Proceeds from the games go to affiliated religious instruction program, thereby reducing parents' tuition costs.

Partner in woodcraft business
  —Initiated, developed and executed own woodcraft business.
  —Coordinated all financial aspects.

PTA membership chairperson
  —Increased membership by 50% over a three-year period.
  —Increased number of parents attending meetings through aggressive telephone campaigns.

Chairperson of church clothing drive
  —Coordinated all efforts of 50 volunteers from collection through distribution.

Education

B.A. candidate, Thomas A. Edison College

A.A. in Dental Hygiene, Fairleigh Dickinson University, May 1970

Personal Data

Health excellent, married, early 40s. Salary negotiable. References on request.

Résumé Review

DO:

- Include a short, concise career objective.
- Include only information that is relevant, to the point, and which supports your objective.
- Use brief phrases rather than sentences to describe what you have done, and start with strong effective action verbs such as supervised, developed, controlled, directed, generated and organized.
- Quantify accomplishments whenever possible. Show the amount of dollars saved or earned, the number of people involved when you reorganized recalls, or how you streamlined operations for greater efficiency and productivity.
- Include courses and affiliations that relate to your career goals.
- Keep personal information to a minimum.
- List educational achievements from college forward.

DO NOT:

- Mention why you left your last job.
- Include previous employers' names and addresses. Say "References furnished on request" at the end of the résumé.
- Include salary history, unless specifically requested.
- Identify marital status, number of children, age (unless you choose to), husband or wife's position, Social Security number, age or weight.

How to Write
A Cover Letter

Why a Cover Letter?

Just as a résumé has one purpose, to get you the interview, so a cover letter has one purpose: to get your résumé read.

When an employer opens the envelope, he or she wants an introductory letter that "covers" why you're sending your résumé. If the cover letter doesn't strike the right note or there are misspellings (especially of his or her name), whiteouts all over the place, or poor grammar, forget about getting your résumé read.

What a cover letter does, in the 15 or so seconds it takes to read it, is create an impression about you. If the impression is negative, the reader will not even glance at your résumé. If the impression is positive, you can be sure your résumé will be read.

What's In It

What's in a cover letter? Just three or four short paragraphs that state 1) why you are writing and sending your résumé, 2) why you are interested in the job, 3) what special quality or experience you have that qualifies you, and 4) your interest in meeting for an interview.

Cover letters cannot be photocopied. They are tailored to specific individuals and must be handled as such. They should be hand-typed on plain white paper, single-spaced, one page only. It's a good idea to include your address and available phone numbers even though you have them on your résumé. (The two items might get separated from each other.)

See the following examples for suggested cover letter styles.

Cover Letter: Example

171 Highway 34
Holmdel, NJ 07733

January 6, 1992

Dr. John Doe
P.O. Box 1000
Matawan, NJ 07747

Dear Dr. Doe:

I am a registered dental hygienist who graduated from the Fones School of Dental Hygiene in Bridgeport, CT this past summer.

Although I am a recent graduate, I have had experience working in a dental office as a dental assistant for over ten years. As you will see from my enclosed résumé, I have extensive experience in both clinical dentistry and office management procedures.

Your advertisement in the Sunday edition of The Asbury Park Press indicates you have a position open for a dental hygienist who wishes to be a member of your health care team. I am interested in applying for that position.

I would appreciate the opportunity to meet with you at your earliest convenience so that we may discuss this further. Please contact me evenings at the number listed below.

Yours truly,

Jane Doe, CDA, RDH
123–4567

Cover Letter: Example

171 Highway 34
Holmdel, NJ 07733

January 6, 1992

Ms. Jane Doe, Regional Sales Mgr.
XYZ Company
72 Madison Ave., Suite 640
New York, NY 10001

Dear Ms. Doe:

Your name was given to me by one of your salespeople, Mr. John Doe, who told me of a sales opening with your company in the New Jersey area.

I am presently employed in a periodontal practice as a clinical dental hygienist, but feel that the challenges and goals of my present position have been met and now wish to pursue a career in sales.

Being a clinical hygienist for seven years has afforded me the opportunity to recommend various home care products such as yours, while expanding my motivational and sales capabilities. This experience has enhanced my ability to be of service to your selling team.

I would welcome the opportunity to discuss with you the possibility of future employment under your direction. Please feel free to contact me any evening at 123/456–7891 so that we may set up an appointment at a time that is convenient for you. My résumé is enclosed.

I look forward to hearing from you.

Sincerely yours,

Jane Doe, RDH, BS

Interviews That Get the Job

Your Interview

For the majority of people, being interviewed is not one of life's most comfortable or enjoyable activities. Even seasoned RDHs claim they still get queasy stomachs at the prospect of the process. When your skills, personality and appearance are being judged, you'd have to be extremely self-confident (or supremely laid back) not to have jangled nerves as you walk through unfamiliar doors.

Here are some guidelines to ease you through that gut-churning time, to glide you through the unknown into the best job situation you could have, whatever your level of experience.

That 10-Second First Impression

The well-worn phrase, "You never have a second chance to make a first impression," rings true during an interview. Be prepared.

When greeting the interviewer, walk confidently toward that person, smile, establish eye contact, and extend a firm, steady handshake.

Women, forget about wearing a uniform or slacks. They're not professional-looking enough. If you don't have a suit or tailored clothes in your wardrobe, opt for a low-keyed dress or matching blouse and skirt of a non-dramatic color and style. Keep your jewelry scaled down. Well-appointed dental offices are quite subdued in color and furnishings. You want to look as if you "fit," not disrupt the environment. Besides, you won't be able to think straight if you're more concerned about how far up your short skirt is climbing or how much noise your bracelets are making. Body language conveys a powerful message.

Men, please note: no jeans, sportshirts, Reeboks. If you don't own a suit, wear a jacket, long-sleeved shirt and tie and matching slacks. If you're going to be taken for "the doctor" anyhow, you might as well look the part. Besides, that's how appealing business and professional men present themselves.

Know Your Values

Before you go on any interview, pinpoint your capabilities. Assess your personality. Define what you want from a job.

Are you looking for personal growth? Professional development? Money? Benefits? Are you a workaholic? Perfectionist? Good team player? What are your career goals and objectives? What is your practice philosophy, your employment expectations? Where are you on infection control? Do you have a clear idea what you want out of a job? Do you know what kind of an environment you want to work in?

You need answers to these questions before you choose any employment situation. Otherwise, you'll end up in any employment situation—not necessarily the one that is best for you.

The American Dental Hygienists' Association suggests RDHs prepare personal philosophies on dental care. Only then, they believe, will both sides be able to discuss the prevailing attitudes, philosophies and treatment modalities with any degree of assurance and concern.

Research Your Market Value

With today's demand for dental hygienists exceeding the supply, you should be armed with what the going pay rate is for entry-level RDHs in your area. Your best sources for this kind of information are your school, your local component of the ADHA, a dental personnel placement agency, or through an anonymous survey conducted by your local association component.

It's up to you to know what your current market value is. How else will you know if what's being offered is fair or not?

Questions to Expect

If you've done your preparation right, you won't be going into an interview blind. You'll be sufficiently prepared to answer any questions asked of you with confidence. The glibbest person on earth cannot answer questions off the cuff without damaging his or her chances of success.

That's the first mistake job-hunters make: attempting to answer questions with virtually no preparation. The second mistake is failing to listen to the question. You annoy the interviewer when you answer a question that wasn't asked or when you give a lot of superfluous information. Keep your ears open as well as your eyes.

Broadly speaking, what employers want to know about you will fall into four categories:

1) Why are you here? (Why do you want to work in *this* place?)
2) What can you do for them? (What are your skills and abilities?)
3) What kind of person are you? (What are your goals, values?)
4) How much are you going to cost them? (What is your salary range and does it fit in with theirs?)

175

Thinking out responses to these categories before an interview will prime you for most questions prospective employers ask.

Questions You Can Ask

You have every right to ask questions to qualify an office. Clarifying expectations on both sides up front, knowing what is expected of you and what you can expect prevents future problems should you decide to take the job.

Here are some topics around which you can frame questions.

1) The normal working day. Ask the interviewer to describe it, including patient load. Ask to look at the appointment book of a typical day. See if the days begin and end at a fixed time and if there are specific times for lunch and breaks. Ask how much time is allotted for each procedure and if it's flexible.

2) Clinical supplies. What are they and who does the ordering?

3) Does the hygienist work while the employer is away from the office (if allowed by state law)?

4) Exactly what are the duties this office expects the dental hygienist to perform? Is there a job description? (Ask to see a copy of it.) If the recall system is involved, is there sufficient administrative time in which to manage it?

5) What is the office philosophy? Is there an office personnel policy manual? How frequently will my performance be measured? By whom?

6) Ask about remuneration, benefits, bonuses, insurance coverage, uniform allowance. Ask about office fees for the procedures you perform.

7) Ask if you can talk to the people with whom you will be working. Your conversations with staff members can give you a sense of the overall "mood" of the office and whether the employees seem happy with their jobs.

The operative phrase here is to be discreet in your timing and the way you phrase your questions. You don't want to come over as demanding or pushy. You simply want information on what's expected of someone in this position.

Evaluate

After the interview, ask yourself: What points did I make that seemed to interest the interviewer? Did I present my qualifications well? Did I overlook any that are pertinent to the position? Did I pass up clues to the best way to "sell" myself? Did I talk too much? Too little? Was I too tense? Too aggressive? Not aggressive enough? Did I maintain eye contact with the interviewer? How can I improve my next interview?

An important question to ask yourself is, "Are there any situations here similar to those that caused me to be unhappy in my last job?" If you have any special concerns along this line, root them out before you agree to anything. If it looks as if there might be a duplication of a negative situation you've previously encountered and found hard to deal with, move on.

Following Up

If you are seriously interested in a job, you'll probably want to go back to the office a second time to nail down the particulars of the job offer. Try to get what was said in writing. It will prevent future misunderstandings and establish a performance standard for you.

You can initiate this document yourself if the office seems too casual or informal in its style to care about generating one. You can say, after you've hammered out what you've agreed upon during discussion, "As I understand it, Doctor, we've agreed to x, y and z. When I go home, I'll put it in written form and bring it back tomorrow. I'd like for us both to sign it." Be non-threatening in your tone; clear, firm and direct in your manner.

Type up a one- or two-page description of your duties, terms, starting date, and salary and benefits as they've been outlined to you and with which you've agreed. Write the letter in your own name, concluding with two lines for both your signatures. Sign your own name and present it to your potential employer for his or hers. Your employer will be greatly impressed by your professionalism and willingness to "start things off on the right foot."

Make your interviews work for you, and when you land a job, it will be the right one.

Resources

Sources of Funding for Education

- GOVERNMENT SOURCES

    Perkins Loans. These are available to both undergraduate and graduate students. Participating schools receive funding from the federal government. The school's financial aid office then distributes the money to applicants meeting eligibility requirements. These can include, along with financial need, the "ability to benefit."

    Stafford Student Loans. These are federally guaranteed student loans made by banks and credit unions. Interest rates are 8 percent for the first four years and 10 percent after that. Upperclassmen can borrow $4,000 a year; graduate students $7,500 per year. Obtain your loan application from a lender and send it for certification to your college.

    Supplemental Loans. Banks provide federally guaranteed loans of up to $4,000 per academic year to students who are not dependents.

    States. Many states have special loan programs for those pursuing careers as teachers, as well as incentives to increase the number of professionals in fields in which the state believes it falls short. These fields are usually medicine, nursing and special and bilingual education.

    Write to the appropriate state department of higher education for data on financial assistance. For addresses, get a copy of *Need a Lift? Educational Opportunities, Careers, Loans, Scholarships, Employment.* Send $2 to the American Legion, Box 1050, Indianapolis, IN 46206. Ask for the latest edition.

    Information about programs administered by the U.S. Department of Education is presented in *The Student Guide to Federal Financial Aid Programs*, which is updated annually. To get a copy, call 800–333–4636 or write Federal Student Aid Programs, P.O. Box 84, Washington, DC 20044.

- FOR WOMEN AND MINORITIES

    Higher Education Opportunities for Minorities and Women, published by the U.S. Department of Education, is a guide to organizations offering assistance. This publication can be found in libraries or may be purchased from the Superintendent of Documents, U.S. Government Printing Office, Washington, DC 20402. Phone 202/783–3238 for price and ordering information.

American Association of University Women (AAUW). This group's Career Development Grants help women who have held a B.A. or other degree for at least five years pay for graduate or professional school. Grants range from $1,000 to $5,000. Applicants must demonstrate that studies will advance their career goals.

This organization has two additional scholarship programs, one of which helps women pursue degrees in fields traditionally closed to them or to finish doctoral or postdoctoral work. The other fellowship helps foreign women to pursue a U.S. education. Contact AAUW Educational Foundation, 1111 16th Street NW, Washington, DC 20036; telephone 202/728-7602.

Clairol Scholarship Program. Clairol makes 50 to 75 annual grants of between $500 and $1,000 to women age 30 or older who have a degree but want to return to school to further their career goals. The foundation also offers the **New York Life Scholarship** for undergraduate studies in the health professions. Contact Clairol Scholarship Program, c/o the Business and Professional Women's Foundation, 2012 Massachusetts Avenue NW, Washington, DC 20036; telephone 202/296-9118.

The Orville Redenbacher Second Start Scholarship Program. This fund assists women entering or returning to undergraduate school. In 1991, twenty $1,000 scholarships were awarded. Applicants must be at least 30 years old. Contact Box 4137, Blair, NE 68009.

The National Dental Association and **Colgate-Palmolive** have joined forces to establish four scholarship programs for black students in dental health. Up to 130 students enrolled in postdoctoral, dental school, dental hygiene and dental assisting education programs will be awarded the scholarships which total $135,000.

The Foundation is offering twenty $500 scholarships to black students who are first-year, full-time dental hygiene students. These will be renewed the following years if the student demonstrates satisfactory progress toward graduation.

For applications or further information, write Dr. Paul Gates, Project Director, NDAF Scholarship Program, P.O. Box 3017, Wayne, NJ 07474, or call 202/244-7555.

- LIBRARY RESOURCES

The following books should be available at your local public or college library. They will give you in-depth information concerning current scholarship, grant and loan programs, many of them from private sources.

181

Lovejoy's Scholarship Guide
Simon & Schuster, Inc.

You Can Win A Scholarship
Barron's Educational Series, Inc.

Scholarships, Fellowships and Loans
Bellman Publishing Co.

How and Where to Get Scholarships and Loans
Simon & Schuster, Inc.

There are other sources of financial aid for education:

- If you are a veteran, tuition assistance may be available through the New G.I. bill. Check with your local VA office.
- Your employer may be able to help with your tuition.
- Many unions provide aid to members and the spouses, sons and daughters of members.
- Most organized religions provide some assistance for members. Ask your religious leader if tuition help is available to you.
- Many local community, civic and fraternal organizations have created scholarship or aid programs. Ask about them.
- **The American Dental Hygienists' Association.**
  Another source of scholastic funding comes from the ADHA's Institute for Oral Health. Through their Institute Scholarship Program, qualified, full-time, entry-level dental hygiene students are eligible for scholarships up to $1,000 through the Procter & Gamble Oral Health/ADHA Institute Scholarship Program.
- The ADHA Institute for Oral Health itself administers scholarships of up to $1500 for full-time dental hygiene students at the certificate/associate, baccalaureate and graduate levels. To qualify, applicants must demonstrate a financial need and have a high GPA. For further information on eligibility requirements, application procedures and deadlines, contact the Institute directly at 312/ 440–8900.

Uniformed Services Dental Facilities

There can be employment opportunities for dental hygienists in a military setting. Jobs for civilians vary, however, since the Uniformed Services train their own people in preventive skills.

The best way to find out is by calling the Personnel Office of the individual facility to ask if there are openings for civilian dental hygienists in the dental clinic.

ALABAMA
US Army Dental Clinic, Redstone Arsenal, Huntsville, AL 35809
US Army Dental Clinic, Fort Rucker, Enterprise, AL 36362
US Army Dental Clinic, Fort McClellan, Anniston, AL 36205
USAF Dental Facility Gunter, Gunter AFB, AL 36114–5300
USAF Dental Clinic Maxwell, Maxwell AFB, AL 36112–5304

ALASKA
US Army Dental Clinic, Fort Richardson, Anchorage, AK 99505
US Army Dental Clinic, Fort Greely, Big Delta, AK 99733
US Army Dental Clinic, Fort Wainwright, Fairbanks, AK 99703
Dental Clinic, 17th Coast Guard District, Juneau, AK 99802
US Coast Guard Support Center Dental Clinic, Kodiak, AK 99619
USAF Dental Clinic, Eielson, Eielson AFB, AK 99702–5300
USAF Dental Clinic, Elmendorf, Elmendorf AFB, AK 99506–5300
US Coast Guard Air Station Dental Clinic, Sitka, AK 99835
Naval Branch Dental Clinic, Adak, FPO Seattle 98791

ARIZONA
US Army Dental Clinic, Fort Huachuca, Sierra Vista, AZ 85613
US Army Dental Clinic, Yuma Proving Ground, Yuma, AZ 85365
USAF Dental Clinic, Davis-Monthan AFB, AZ 85707–5300
USAF Dental Clinic, Luke AFB, AZ 85309–5300

USAF Dental Clinic, Williams AFB, AZ 85240–5300
Naval Branch Dental Clinic, MCAS Yuma, AZ 85369

ARKANSAS
US Army Dental Clinic, Pine Bluff Arsenal, Pine Bluff*
(Mailing address: Reynolds Army Community Hospital, Fort Sill, Lawton, OK 73503–6400)
US Army Dental Clinic, Fort Chaffee, Fort Smith*
(Mailing address: Reynolds Army Community Hospital, Fort Sill, Lawton, OK 73503–6400)
USAF Dental Clinic, Blytheville AFB, AR 72315–5300
USAF Dental Clinic, Little Rock, AR 72099–5300

*Dental clinic closed several months annually.

CALIFORNIA
US Army Dental Clinic, Sierra Army Depot, Herlong, CA 96113
US Army Dental Clinic, Fort Hunter Liggett, Jolon, CA 93928
US Army Dental Clinic, Presidio of Monterey, Monterey, CA 93940
US Army Dental Clinic, Fort Irwin, Barstow, CA 92310
US Coast Guard Dental Clinic, Base Terminal Island, Long Beach, CA 90822
USAF Dental Clinic Los Angeles, Los Angeles AFS, CA 90009–5300
USAF Dental Clinic Norton, Norton AFB, CA 92409–5300
USAF Dental Clinic McClellan, McClellan AFB, CA 95652–5300
USAF Dental Clinic Beale, Beale AFB, CA 95903–5300

USAF Dental Clinic Castle, Castle AFB, CA
95342–5300
USAF Dental Clinic Edwards, Edwards AFB,
CA 93523–5300
USAF Dental Clinic George, George AFB, CA
92392–5300
USAF Dental Clinic March, March AFB, CA
92518–5300
USAF Dental Clinic Travis, Travis AFB, CA
94535–5300
USAF Dental Clinic Vandenberg, Vandenberg
AFB, CA 93437–5300
USAF Dental Clinic Mather, Mather AFB, CA
95655–5300
Navy Dental Clinics:
San Diego, CA 92136–5147
Camp Pendleton, CA 92055–5009
Long Beach, CA 90822–5096
San Francisco, CA 94130–5030
Naval Branch Dental Clinics:
CBC, Port Hueneme, CA 93043
FLEASWTRACENPAC, San Diego, CA
92147
MCAGC, Twentynine Palms, CA 92278
El Toro, Santa Ana, CA 92709
MCAS, H Tustin, CA 92710
MCMWTC, Bridgeport, CA 93517
MCRD, San Diego, CA 92140
NAS, Alameda, CA 94501
NAS, Lemoore, CA 93245
NAS, Miramar, San Diego, CA 92145
NAS, Moffett Field, CA 94035
NAS, North Island, San Diego, CA 23460
NAS, Point Mugu, CA 93042
NAVCOMSTA, Stockton, CA 95203
NAVPGSCOL, Monterey, CA 93943
NAVPHIBASE, Coronado, CA 92155
NAVSTA, Mare Island, CA 94592
NAVWPNCEN, China Lake, CA 93555
NSC, San Diego, CA 92132
NTC, San Diego, CA 92133
SUBASE, San Diego, CA 92106
WPNSTA, Concord, CA 94520
WPNSTA, Seal Beach, CA 90740
MCLB, Barstow, CA 92311
NAF, El Centro, CA 92243

COLORADO
US Army Dental Clinic, Fitzsimons, Aurora,
CO 80045–5000
US Army Dental Clinic, Fort Carson, Colorado
Springs, CO 80913-5000

USAF Dental Clinic Lowry, Lowry AFB, CO
80230–5300
USAF Dental Clinic Peterson, Peterson AFB,
CO 80914–5300
USAF Academy Dental Clinic, USAFA,
Colorado Springs, CO 80840-5300

CONNECTICUT
Branch Naval Dental Clinic, SUBASE New
London, Groton, CT 06340

DELAWARE
USAF Dental Clinic Dover, Dover AFB, DE
19902–5300

DISTRICT OF COLUMBIA
US Army Dental Clinic, Walter Reed,
Washington, DC 20307–5000
US Army Dental Clinic, Fort McNair,
Washington, DC 20319
US Army Dental Clinic, Pentagon,
Washington, DC 20310
USAF Dental Clinic Bolling, Bolling AFB, DC
20332–5300
Naval Branch Dental Clinics:
NAF, Washington, DC 20390
NAVSECSTA, Washington, DC 20390
Navy Yard, Washington, DC 20374
Arlington Annex, Washington, DC 20370
Marine Barracks, 8th & I, Washington, DC
20390

FLORIDA
USAF Dental Clinic Eglin, Eglin AFB, FL
32542–5300
USAF Dental Clinic Homestead, Homestead
AFB, FL 33039–5300
USAF Dental Clinic MacDill, MacDill AFB, FL
33609–5300
USAF Dental Clinic Patrick, Patrick AFB, FL
32925–5300
USAF Dental Clinic Tyndall, Tyndall AFB, FL
32403–5300
US Coast Guard Base Dental Clinic, 100
MacArthur Causeway, Miami Beach, FL
33139
US Coast Guard Air Station Dental Clinic,
Clearwater, FL 33520
Navy Dental Clinics:
Jacksonville, FL 32212-0074
Orlando, FL 32813–6400
Pensacola, FL 32508–5800

Naval Branch Dental Clinics:
  NAS, Cecil Field, FL 32215
  NAS, Key West, FL 33040
  NAS, Whiting Field, Milton, FL 32570
  NAVCOASTSYSCEN, Panama City, FL
    32407
  NAVSTA, Mayport, FL 32228
  NAVTECHTRACEN, Pensacola, FL 32511

GEORGIA

US Army Dental Clinic, Fort Gordon, Augusta,
  GA 30905–5060
US Army Dental Clinic, Fort Benning,
  Columbus, GA 31905
US Army Dental Clinic, Fort Stewart,
  Savannah, GA 31314–5300
US Army Dental Clinic, Hunter Army Airfield,
  Savannah, GA 31409
US Army Dental Clinic, Fort McPherson,
  Atlanta, GA 30330
USAF Dental Clinic, 347 Medical Group,
  Moody AFB, GA 31601–5300
USAF Dental Clinic, Robins AFB, GA 31098–
  5300
Naval Branch Dental Clinics:
  MCLB, Albany, GA 31704
  NAS, Atlanta, Marietta, GA 30060
  NAVSCSCOL, Athens, GA 30601

HAWAII

US Army Dental Clinic, Tripler, Honolulu, Oahu
  (Mailing address: Tripler Army Medical
    Center, HI 96853–5300)
US Army Dental Clinic, Schofield Barracks,
  Honolulu, Oahu
  (Mailing address: Tripler Army Medical
    Center, HI 96853–5300)
US Army Dental Clinic, Fort Shafter, Honolulu,
  Oahu
  (Mailing address: Tripler Army Medical
    Center, HI 96853–5300)
US Army Dental Clinic, Pohakuloa Training
  Center, Hilo, Hawaii
  (Mailing address: Tripler Army Medical
    Center, HI 96853–5300)
USAF Dental Clinic Hickam, Hickam AFB, HI
  96853–5300
US Coast Guard Base Dental Clinic, Honolulu,
  Oahu, HI 96819
Naval Dental Clinic, Pearl Harbor, Oahu, HI
  96860

Naval Branch Dental Clinics:
  MCAS, Kaneohe Bay, HI 96863
  NAS, Barbers Point, HI 96862
  NAVCAMS, Eastpac, Wahiawa, HI 96786
  NAVMAG, Lualualei, HI 96792
  MCB Camp H.M. Smith, HI 96861
  PACMISRNG Kekaha Kauai, HI 96752

IDAHO

USAF Dental Clinic Mountain Home, Mountain
  Home AFB, ID 83648–300
Naval Branch Dental Clinic, Idaho Falls, ID
  83402

ILLINOIS

US Army Dental Clinic, Fort Sheridan,
  Highwood, IL 60037
USAF Dental Clinic, Scott AFB, IL 62225–
  5300
USAF Dental Clinic, Chanute AFB, IL 61868–
  5300Naval Branch Dental Clinic, NAS,
  Glenview, IL 60026Naval Dental Clinic,
  Great Lakes, IL 60088–5258

INDIANA

USAF Dental Clinic Grissom, Grissom AFB, IN
  46971–5300
US Army Dental Clinic, Fort Benjamin
  Harrison, Indianapolis, IN 46216–7000

KANSAS

US Army Dental Clinic, Fort Leavenworth,
  Leavenworth, KS 66027-5400
US Army Dental Clinic, Fort Riley, Junction
  City, KS 66442–5036
USAF Dental Clinic McConnell, McConnell
  AFB, KS 67221–5300

KENTUCKY

US Army Dental Clinic, Fort Campbell,
  Hopkinsville, KY 42223
US Army Dental Clinic, Fort Knox,
  Elizabethtown, KY 40121

LOUISIANA

US Army Dental Clinic, Fort Polk, Leesville, LA
  71459
USAF Dental Clinic, Barksdale AFB, LA
  71110–5300
USAF Dental Clinic, England AFB, LA 71311–
  5300
Naval Branch Dental Clinic, NAVSUPPACT,
  New Orleans, LA 70146

MAINE

USAF Dental Clinic, Loring, Loring AFB, ME 04751-5300
Naval Branch Dental Clinics:
NAS, Brunswick, ME 04011
NAVCOMMU, Cutler, East Machias, ME 04630
NAVSECGRUACT, Winter Harbor, ME 04693

MARYLAND

US Army Dental Clinic, Fort Meade, Odenton, MD 20755
US Army Dental Clinic, Fort Richie, Cascade, MD 21719
US Army Dental Clinic, Edgewood Area, Aberdeen Proving Ground, MD 21005
US Army Dental Clinic, Fort Detrick, Frederick, MD 21701
USAF Dental Clinic Andrews, Andrews AFB, MD 20331-5300
Naval Dental Clinic, Bethesda, MD 20814
Naval Branch Dental Clinics:
NAS, Patuxent River, MD 20670
NAVORDSTA, Indian Head, MD 20640
USNA, Annapolis, MD 21402

MASSACHUSETTS

US Army Dental Clinic, Fort Devens, Ayer, MA 01433
USAF Dental Clinic Hanscom, Hanscom AFB, MA 01730-5300
Naval Branch Dental Clinic, South Weymouth, MA 02190

MICHIGAN

USAF Dental Clinic K.I. Sawyer, K.I. Sawyer AFB, MI 49843-5300
USAF Dental Clinic Wurtsmith, Wurtsmith AFB, MI 48753-5300
Naval Branch Dental Clinic, NAF, Detroit, MI 48043

MISSISSIPPI

USAF Dental Clinic, Columbus AFB, MS 39701-5300
USAF Dental Clinic, Keesler AFB, MS 39534-5300
Naval Branch Dental Clinics:
CBC, Gulfport, MS 39501
Naval Home, Gulfport, MS 39501
NAS, Meridian, MS 39309
SUBSHIP Pascagoula, MS 39567

MISSOURI

US Army Dental Clinic, Fort Leonard Wood, Waynesville, MO 65473
US Army Dental Clinic, Federal Building, 1520 Market St., St. Louis, MO 63103
USAF Dental Clinic Whiteman, Whiteman AFB, MO 65301-5300
Naval Branch Dental Clinic, Marine Corps Finance Center, Kansas City, MO 64197

MONTANA

USAF Dental Clinic Malmstrom, Malmstrom AFB, MT 59402-5300

NEBRASKA

USAF Dental Clinic Offutt, Offutt AFB, NE 68113-5300

NEVADA

US Army Dental Clinic, Hawthorne Army Ammunition Depot, Hawthorne
(Mailing address: Letterman Army Medical Center, Presidio of SF, CA 94129-6700)
USAF Dental Clinic Nellis, Nellis AFB, NV 89191-5300
Naval Branch Dental Clinic, NAS, Fallon, NV 89406

NEW HAMPSHIRE

509 Strategic Hospital, Pease AFB, NH 03803-5300
Naval Branch Dental Clinic, NAVSHIPYD, Portsmouth, NH 03801

NEW JERSEY

US Army Dental Clinic, Fort Dix, Pemberton, NJ 08640
US Army Dental Clinic, Fort Monmouth, Eatontown, NJ 07703
USAF Clinic McGuire, McGuire AFB, NJ 08641-5300
US Coast Guard Training Center Clinic, Cape May, NJ 08204
Naval Branch Dental Clinic, NAVAIRENGCEN, Lakehurst, NJ 08733

NEW MEXICO

US Army Dental Clinic, White Sands Missile Range, Las Cruces
(Mailing address: William Beaumont Army Medical Center, El Paso, TX 79920-5001)
USAF Dental Clinic, 27 Medical Group, Cannon AFB, NM 88101-5300

USAF Dental Clinic, Holloman, Holloman AFB, NM 88330-5300

USAF Dental Clinic, Kirtland AFB, NM 87117-5300

NEW YORK

US Army Dental Clinic, US Military Academy, West Point, NY 10996

US Army Dental Clinic, Fort Hamilton, Brooklyn, NY 11252

US Army Dental Clinic, Seneca Army Depot, Romulus, NY 14541

US Army Dental Clinic, Fort Drum, Watertown, NY 13601

US Coast Guard Support Center Clinic, Governors Island, New York City, NY 10004

Naval Branch Dental Clinic, NAVSTA New York, Brooklyn, NY 11251

Naval Branch Dental Clinic, NAVADMINUNIT, Ballston Spa, NY 12020

USAF Dental Clinic, Griffiss AFB, NY 13441-5300

USAF Dental Clinic, Plattsburgh AFB, NY 12903-5300

NORTH CAROLINA

US Army Dental Clinic, Fort Bragg, Fayetteville, NC 28307-5000

USAF Dental Clinic, Pope AFB, NC 28308-5300

USAF Dental Clinic, Seymour Johnson AFB, NC 27531-5300

US Coast Guard Group Dental Clinic Fort Macon, Atlantic Beach, NC US Coast Guard Marine Safety Office Dental Clinic, Wilmington, NC 28401-3907

Naval Dental Clinic, Camp Lejeune, NC 28542

Naval Branch Dental Clinics:
MCAS Cherry Point, NC 28533
MCAS Jacksonville, NC 28545

NORTH DAKOTA

USAF Dental Clinic, 321 Strategic Hospital, Grand Forks AFB, ND 58205-5300

USAF Dental Clinic, 91 Strategic Hospital, Minot AFB, ND 58705-5300

OHIO

USAF Dental Clinic Wright-Patterson, Wright-Patterson AFB, OH 45433-5300

OKLAHOMA

US Army Dental Clinic, Fort Sill, Lawton, OK 73503

USAF Dental Clinic, Vance AFB, OK 73701-5300

USAF Dental Clinic, Altus AFB, OK 73521-5300

USAF Dental Clinic, Tinker AFB, OK 73145-5300

OREGON

US Coast Guard Air Station Dental Clinic, 2000 Connecticut Avenue, North Bend, OR 97459

PENNSYLVANIA

US Army Dental Clinic, Carlisle Barracks, Carlisle, PA 17013

Naval Dental Clinic, Philadelphia, PA 19112

Naval Branch Dental Clinic, NAS, Willow Grove, PA 19090

RHODE ISLAND

Naval Dental Clinics:
Newport, RI 02841
NAVSUBBASE New London, Groton, CT 06340

SOUTH CAROLINA

US Army Dental Clinic, Fort Jackson, Columbia, SC 29207

USAF Dental Clinic, Charleston AFB, SC 29404-5300

USAF Dental Clinic, 354 Medical Group, Myrtle Beach AFB, SC 29577-5300

USAF Dental Clinic, 363 Medical Group, Shaw AFB, SC 29152-5300

Naval Dental Clinics:
Parris Island, SC 29905
Charleston, SC 29408

Naval Branch Dental Clinic, WPNSTA Charleston, SC 29408

SOUTH DAKOTA

44 Strategic Hospital, Ellsworth AFB, SD 57706-5300

TENNESSEE

Naval Branch Dental Clinic, Millington, TN 38054

TEXAS

US Army Dental Clinic, Fort Bliss, El Paso, TX 79916

US Army Dental Clinic, Fort Hood, Killeen, TX 76544

US Army Dental Clinic, Fort Sam Houston, San Antonio, TX 78234

USAF Dental Clinic, Brooks AFB, TX 78235–5300

USAF Dental Clinic, Goodfellow AFB, TX 76908–5300

USAF Dental Clinic, Kelly AFB, TX 78241–5300

USAF Dental Clinic, Randolph AFB, TX 78150–5300

USAF Dental Clinic, Bergstrom AFB, TX 78743–5300

USAF Dental Clinic, Carswell AFB, TX 76127–5300

USAF Dental Clinic, Dyess AFB, TX 79607–5300

USAF Dental Clinic, Lackland AFB, TX 78236–5300

USAF Dental Clinic, Laughlin AFB, TX 78843–5300

USAF Dental Clinic, Reese AFB, TX 79489–5300

USAF Dental Clinic, Sheppard AFB, Tx 76311–5300

Naval Branch Dental Clinic:
  NAS, Chase Field, Beeville, TX 78103
  NAS, Dallas, TX 75211
  NAS, Kingsville, TX 78363
  NAS, Corpus Christi, TX 78419

UTAH

US Army Dental Clinic, Dugway Proving Ground, Dugway
  (Mailing address: Fitzsimons Army Medical Center, Aurora, CO 80045–5000)
  USAF Dental Clinic Hill, Hill AFB, UT 84056–5300

VIRGINIA

US Army Dental Clinic, Defense General Supply Center, Richmond, VA 23219

US Army Dental Clinic, Fort A.P. Hill, Bowling Green
  (Mailing address: Dewitt Army Hospital, Fort Belvoir, VA 22060–5166)

US Army Dental Clinic, Vint Hill Farms Station, Warrenton
  (Mailing address: Dewitt Army Hospital, Fort Belvoir, VA 22060–5166)

US Army Dental Clinic, Fort Belvoir, Springfield, VA 22060–5166

US Army Dental Clinic, Fort Monroe, Hampton
  (Mailing address: McDonald Army Hospital, Fort Eustis, VA 23604–5567)

US Army Dental Clinic, Fort Story

  (Mailing address: McDonald Army Hospital, Fort Eustis, VA 23604–5567)

US Army Dental Clinic, Fort Eustis, Lee Hall
  (Mailing address: McDonald Army Hospital, Fort Eustis, VA 23604–5567)

US Army Dental Clinic, Fort Lee, Petersburg, VA 23801–5260

US Army Dental Clinic, Fort Myer, Arlington, VA 22211

US Army Dental Clinic, Fort Pickett, Blackstone, VA 23824

USAF Dental Clinic Langley, Langley AFB, VA 23665–5300

Naval Dental Clinic, Norfolk, VA 23511

Naval Branch Dental Clinics:
  MCDEC, Quantico, VA 22134
  NAS, Oceana, Virginia Beach, VA 23460
  NAVSHIPYD, Portsmouth, VA 23700
  SUPSHIP, Newport News, VA 23607
  WPNSTA, Yorktown, VA 23691
  NAVPHIBASE, Little Creek, Norfolk, VA 23521
  NAVSWC, Dahlgren, VA 22443
  FCTC Dam Neck, Virginia Beach, VA 23461
  CINCLANTFLT, Norfolk, VA 23511
  Armed Forces Staff College, Norfolk, VA 23511

WASHINGTON

US Army Dental Clinic, Fort Lewis, Tacoma, WA 98433

USAF Dental Clinic McChord, McChord AFB, WA 98438–5300

USAF Dental Clinic Fairchild, Fairchild AFB, WA 99011–5300

Makah Air Force Station, Neah Bay, WA 98357

Naval Dental Clinic, Bremerton, WA 98314–5245

Naval Branch Dental Clinics:
  NAS, Whidbey Island, Oak Harbor, WA 98278
  SUBASE Bangor, Bremerton, WA 98315–5245
  NAVFAC Pacific Beach, WA 98115
  NAVSTA Seattle, WA 98115

WISCONSIN

US Army Dental Clinic, Fort McCoy, Sparta, WI 54656*

*Closed several months each year.

WYOMING

USAF Dental Clinic F.E. Warren, F.E. Warren AFB, WY 82005–5300

Veterans Administration Hospital Locations

VA hospitals at the following locations range in capacity from approximately 100 to over 1,500 beds. Average bed capacity is about 600. Most have general medical and surgical, pulmonary disease, and psychiatric units. Others are predominantly psychiatric. Many have research programs, dental clinics, outpatient clinics or domiciliaries. Contact the Personnel Officer at the individual hospital for specific information on jobs.

ALABAMA
Birmingham 35233
Montgomery 36109
Tuscaloosa 35404
Tuskegee 36083

ALASKA
Anchorage 99501

ARIZONA
Phoenix 85012
Prescott 86301
Tucson 85723

ARKANSAS
Fayetteville 72702
Little Rock 72206

CALIFORNIA
Fresno 93703
Livermore 94550
Loma Linda 92357
Long Beach 90822
Los Angeles (West Los Angeles) 90073
Martinez 94553
Palo Alto 94304
San Diego 92161
San Francisco 94121
Sepulveda 91343

COLORADO
Denver 80220
Fort Lyon 81038
Grand Junction 81501

CONNECTICUT
Newington 06111
West Haven 06516

DELAWARE
Wilmington 19805

DISTRICT OF COLUMBIA
Washington 20422

FLORIDA
Bay Pines 33504
Gainesville 32602
Lake City 32055
Miami 33125
Tampa 33612

GEORGIA
Augusta 30910
Decatur 30033
Dublin 31021

HAWAII
Honolulu 96813

IDAHO
Boise 83702

ILLINOIS
Chicago (Lakeside) 60611
Chicago (West Side) 60680
Danville 61832
North Chicago 60064
Hines 60141
Marion 62959

INDIANA
Fort Wayne 46805
Indianapolis 46202
Marion 46952

IOWA
Des Moines 50310
Iowa City 52240
Knoxville 50138

KANSAS
Leavenworth 66048
Topeka 66622
Wichita 67211

KENTUCKY
Lexington 40511
Louisville 40202

LOUISIANA
Alexandria 71301
New Orleans 70146
Shreveport 71130

MAINE
Togus 04330

MARYLAND
Baltimore 21218
Fort Howard 21052
Perry Point 21902

MASSACHUSETTS
Bedford 01730
Boston 02130
Brockton/West Roxbury 02401
Northamptom 01060

MICHIGAN
Allen Park 48101
Ann Arbor 48105
Iron Mountain 49801
Saginaw 48602

MINNESOTA
Minneapolis 55417
St. Cloud 56301

MISSISSIPPI
Biloxi 39531
Jackson 39216

MISSOURI
Columbia 65201
Kansas City 64128
Poplar Bluff 63901
St. Louis 63125

MONTANA
Ft. Harrison 59636
Miles City 59301

NEBRASKA
Grand Island 68801
Lincoln 68510
Omaha 68105

NEVADA
Reno 89520

NEW HAMPSHIRE
Manchester 03104

NEW JERSEY
East Orange 07019
Lyons 07939

NEW MEXICO
Albuquerque 87108

NEW YORK
Albany 12208
Batavia 14020
Bath 14810
Bronx 10468
Brooklyn 11209
Buffalo 14215
Canandaigua 14424
Castle Point 12511
Montrose 10548
New York 10010
Northport (Long Island) 11768
Syracuse 13210

NORTH CAROLINA
Asheville 28805
Durham 27705
Fayetteville 28301
Salisbury 28144

NORTH DAKOTA
Fargo 58102

OHIO
Chillicothe 45601
Cincinnati 45520
Cleveland 44109
Dayton 45428

OKLAHOMA
Muskogee 74401
Oklahoma City 73104

OREGON
Portland 97207
Roseburg 97470

PENNSYLVANIA
Altoona 16603
Butler 16001
Coatesville 19320
Erie 16501
Lebanon 17042
Philadelphia 19104
Pittsburgh (Highland Dr.) 15206
Pittsburg (University Dr. C) 15240
Wilkes-Barre 18711

PUERTO RICO
San Juan 96528

RHODE ISLAND
Providence 02908

190

SOUTH CAROLINA
Charleston 29403
Columbia 29201

SOUTH DAKOTA
Fort Meade 57741
Hot Springs 57747
Sioux Falls 57101

TENNESSEE
Memphis 38104
Mountain Home (Johnson City) 37601
Murfreesboro 37130
Nashville 37203

TEXAS
Amarillo 79106
Big Springs 79720
Bonham 75418
El Paso 79925
Dallas 75216
Houston 77211
Kerrville 78028
Marlin 76661
San Antonio 78284
Temple 76501
Waco 76703

UTAH
Salt Lake City 84148

VERMONT
White River Jct. 05001

VIRGINIA
Hampton 23667
Richmond 23249
Salem 24153

WASHINGTON
American Lake, Tacoma 98493
Seattle 98108
Spokane 99208
Walla Walla 99362

WEST VIRGINIA
Beckley 25801
Clarksburg 26301
Huntington 25701
Martinsburg 25401

WISCONSIN
Madison 53705
Tomah 54660
Wood (Milwaukee) 53193

WYOMING
Cheyenne 82001
Sheridan 82801

Appendix

Degree Completion Programs

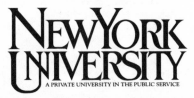
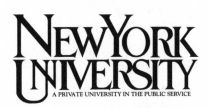

BALTIMORE COLLEGE OF DENTAL SURGERY
DENTAL SCHOOL
UNIVERSITY OF MARYLAND AT BALTIMORE

ARE YOU SEEKING RENEWED ENTHUSIASM FOR DENTAL HYGIENE PRACTICE AND NEW CAREER OPTIONS?

Degree Completion Bachelor of Science and Master of Science program can prepare you for positions in:

- Administration
- Education
- Community/Institutional Health
- Clinical Practice
- Management
- Research

Why the University of Maryland?

- Individually tailored program
- Career oriented practicums
- Full or part-time schedules
- Reasonable tuition
- Work opportunities and financial aid
- Nationally recognized faculty
- Atmosphere of caring and excellence
- Baltimore – a renaissance city

Department of Dental Hygiene
666 W. Baltimore Street, Baltimore, Maryland 21201
410/328-7773

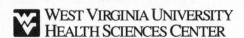

WEST VIRGINIA UNIVERSITY
HEALTH SCIENCES CENTER

Specializing in Unique Educational Programs in Dental Hygiene

Four-Year Integrated Bachelor of Science in Dental Hygiene	Degree Completion Bachelor of Science in Dental Hygiene	Master of Science in Dental Hygiene

- **Curricular Options in:**
  Education / Administration
  Advanced Clinical
  Research
  Special Patient Care
  Advanced Dental Science
  Office Management

- **Excellent Tuition**

- **Full or Part-time Enrollment**

- **August or January Admittance**

CONTACT: Dr. Christina B. DeBiase, Coordinator
Degree Completion and Master of
Science Programs
Mrs. Barbara K. Komives, Chairperson
Integrated Program
West Virginia University
Department of Dental Hygiene
1073 Health Sciences Building North
Morgantown, West Virginia 26506
(304) 293-3417

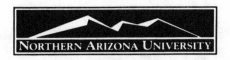

Hygiene Supporters

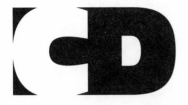

**Career Directions Press thanks
the following advertisers
for their support...**

Colgate-Palmolive Company

Dental Power Services, Inc.

Oral-B Laboratories

Procter & Gamble

Warner-Lambert Company

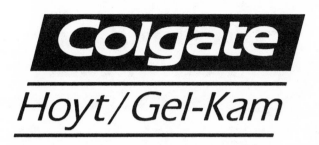

Hoyt/Gel-Kam

Dedicated to supporting the Dental Hygiene Community by offering quality Therapy Products as well as career alternatives.

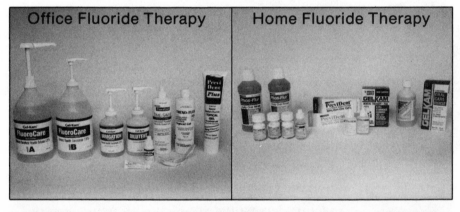

Office Fluoride Therapy   Home Fluoride Therapy

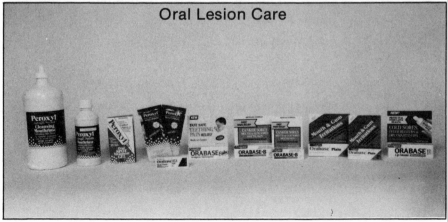

Oral Lesion Care

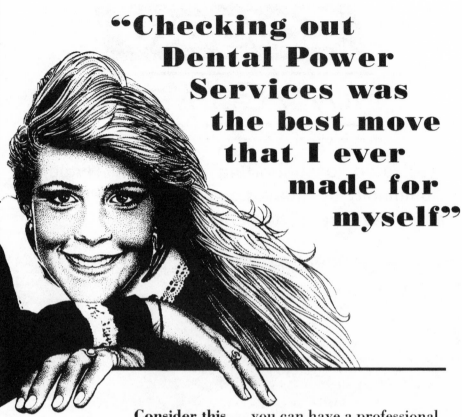

"Checking out Dental Power Services was the best move that I ever made for myself"

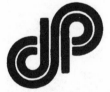

Consider this ... you can have a professional hygiene position working in a military dental facility, providing yourself with paid vacation, paid holidays, paid sick leave, and our company profit sharing program.

Check us out ... the leading provider of hygiene services to the U.S. Government. Call Dental Power Services today ...

804/873-3371

751-K Thimble Shoals Boulevard, Newport News, Virginia 23606

Dental Power Services, Inc.

RECOMMEND FOR EASIER PROPHYS

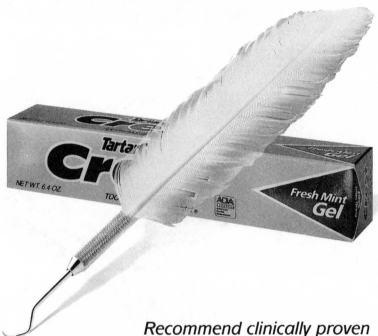

Recommend clinically proven Tartar Control Crest and give you and your patients the advantage of easier prophys.

Recommend

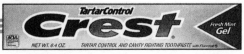

Helps keep brushing and flossing effective

THE ORAL-B TOOTHBRUSH W
SUPERIOR, END-ROUNDED BF

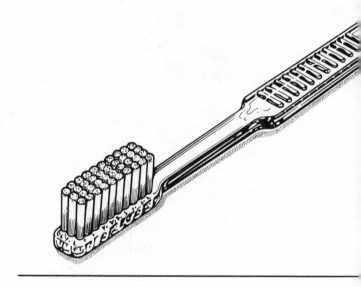

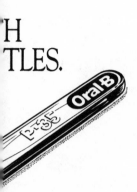
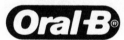

It's Clear Which Mouthrinse Is ADA-Accepted to Help
Fight Plaque and Gingivitis...

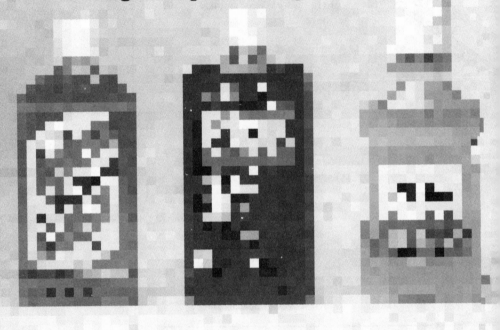

LISTERINE® ANTISEPTIC

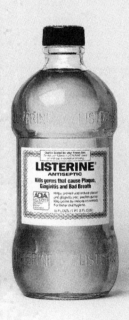

Listerine Is Accepted by the ADA Council on Dental Therapeutics to Help Prevent Supragingival Plaque and Gingivitis*[1]

"Listerine has been shown to help prevent and reduce supragingival plaque accumulation and gingivitis when used in a conscientiously applied program of oral hygiene and regular professional care. Its effect on periodontitis has not been determined."

Council on Dental Therapeutics
American Dental Association

ACCEPTED
American
Dental
Association

Reference:
1. Council on Dental Therapeutics Accepts Listerine. *JADA* 117: 515-516, 1988.
*When used as a supplement to daily oral hygiene and regular professional care.

...First-line antimicrobial defense for your patients.

ORDER FORM

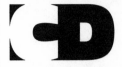

CAREER DIRECTIONS
for Dental Hygienists

Your Guide to Change and Opportunity
By REGINA DREYER THOMAS, RDH

☐ YES!

Please rush a copy of this unique publication to the address below. Enclosed is my check or money order for $19.00 ($16.50 for book plus $2.50 for shipping and handling) made out to CAREER DIRECTIONS PRESS. I understand that if I am not satisfied with the book I can return it within two weeks of receipt for a full refund. (NJ residents please add appropriate sales tax. Thank you.)

Please print clearly

Name _____

Address_____

City _____

State _____ Zip _____

Offer valid in U.S. only.
Allow at least three weeks for delivery.

Mail Order Form and Check or Money Order to:

Career Directions Press
171 Highway 34
Holmdel, NJ 07733

REGINA DREYER THOMAS, RDH, BS, MPA

Ms. Thomas brings with her an extensive background in both the dental profession and dental industry. She has

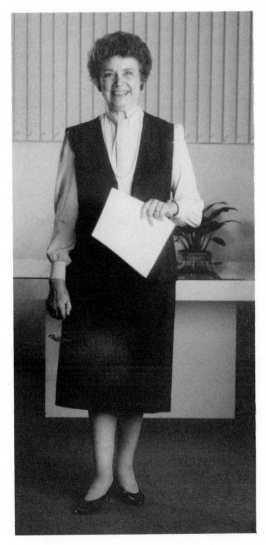

served as director of training for a dental manufacturer, supervisor of a dental clinic in a large metropolitan hospital, been an assistant professor in a school of dental hygiene, a school dental hygienist and both an RDH and dental assistant in private practice.

Her present career centers around her publishing company, **Career Directions Press**, dental academia and industry consulting. She is a consulting editor for *RDH* magazine and lectures on career development to practicing dental hygienists.

Ms. Thomas holds a B.S. in health education and a master's degree in public administration. She is a member of the ADHA and other professional organizations.